MEDICAL TERMINOLOGY

JERRY S. FINDLEY

ABSORPTION
LYMPHATIC SYSTEM
VESSELS
MUSCULAR
SKELETAL SYSTEM
GLANDS
ELECTROPHYSIOLOGY
ENDOCRINE
ANXIETY
TENDONS
ACCESSORY
BLADDER
AFFECTIVE
AXIAL AND APPENDICULAR SKELETON
SYMPATHETIC
INTESTINES
FUNCTIONS
UPPER DIGESTIVE SYSTEM
IMMUNE SYSTEM
KIDNEYS
BURNS
CARDIOVASCULAR
FEMALE URINARY
PHARMACOLOGY
STOMACH
PARASYMPATHETIC
MUSCLES
DISORDERS
BLOOD AND LYMPH
MENTAL HEALTH
BLOOD TYPES
LOWER NERVOUS BRAIN
ELIMINATION
PERSONALITY
ABSORPTION
HEART
INTEGUMENTARY
ADMINISTRATION
WHITE BLOOD CELLS
COMPONENTS OF BLOOD
METABOLIZING
MALE URINARY
DIGESTIVE
RESPIRATORY
PANCREAS
SPINAL CORD
LOWER NERVOUS BRAIN
RED BLOOD CELLS
JOINTS
NERVES
URINARY
DISORDERS

Kendall Hunt
publishing company

Kendall Hunt
publishing company

www.kendallhunt.com
Send all inquiries to:
4050 Westmark Drive
Dubuque, IA 52004-1840

ISBN 978-1-5249-2101-9

Published in the United States of America

Dedication

This book would not have been possible without the support and encouragement from my family to step out and finally give it a try. Tina, Ashlea, Tyler, and Alyson; thanks for taking this journey with me.

Contents

CHAPTER 1

Intro to Med Term

Medical terminology is the study of terms. These terms are used in various medical disciplines. As society and medicine have progressed so too has the use of medical terms. Medical terms are used daily and our ability to use those words in the proper context is paramount to us to begin to be good practitioners. It takes a good knowledge and understanding of medical terminology to navigate the medical profession.

Medical terminology is rooted in Greek and Latin. There are 1200 Greek and Latin root words that will make up more than 15,000 medical terms that we utilize. With Greek and Latin being the root medical terminology, it makes the study of these terms universal. People from different countries and languages have a common thread when documenting and speaking these terms. For us to be able to consistently and accurately describe a word we must be able to break a word down to its simplest form to be able to define it. No matter that length of the word (esophagogastroduodenoscopy) we must break the word down and figure out its meaning. To do that we must go all the way back to English class to refresh ourselves on prefixes, suffixes, and root words. This foundation will enable us to understand each body system.

Latin	Greek
lingu/o = tongue	gloss/o = tongue
bilingual	glossary
sublingual	glossitis

Notice the first term under the column heading Latin, "bilingual." It means pertaining to two languages. This term is very common in that when we hear of someone being bilingual, we know that they are able to speak more than one language. Sublingual is a medical term. Sub means under, with the suffix al meaning pertaining to. This term means pertaining to under the tongue. If we give a medication by a sublingual route, we are giving the medication under the tongue. One of the most common medications that we give sublingually is nitroglycerin. This medication dissolves very quickly when given sublingually and quickly transitions into the bloodstream.

The first term under the column heading Greek is gloss/o, also meaning tongue. Glossitis is a medical term meaning inflammation of the tongue. The suffix -itis means inflammation. This is a very common term to describe swelling. For someone having an allergic reaction from eating can have glossitis.

There are around 90% of healthcare terms that can be built from word parts. The other 10% are not and examples of those are cataract and asthma. When describing general medical terms, we use diagnosis, prognosis, acute, chronic, sign, and symptom. For medical professionals to have a good grasp on medical terminology and the ability to convey information, we must be knowledgeable in these basic terms. Diagnosis is the present condition. Dia means through or complete and -gnosis means a state of knowledge. Literally the term diagnosis means a complete state of knowledge. You go to the physician because you have a cold and the physician gets a complete state of knowledge of your condition using his or her evaluation of the signs, symptoms, and history. This is a present condition that is usually treated with an antibiotic for a short period of time and your infection clears up and you feel better. A prognosis is a future condition. Pro means before or in front of and gnosis means state of knowledge. A prognosis is a state of knowledge ahead of time, so the physician is predicting ahead of time based on his or her knowledge of what the outcome will be. You go the physician, and he or she tells you that you have a serious disease and the prognosis is poor. In other words, the disease in hard to treat and the outcome is serious or fatal. An acute disease is short-term/sudden onset and sharp. A person is walking and suddenly has acute chest pain—meaning the pain had a sudden onset and was sharp. A chronic disease is long term and returns. A person that has arthritis has a disease that is long term and returns. This person will have this condition for the rest of his or her life. While there may be medications to help with a chronic disease, it will always be there and will return. In medical terms, an instrument used to measure time is a chronometer or your watch! When we go and see the physician, we give his or her a list of things that are wrong with us. The physician separates this list into two categories: signs and symptoms. A sign is objective, and it can be seen and/or measured. A sign is something that we can see or feel. If you tell the physician you have a fever, or a rash, or you have blisters, you are giving the physician a sign. A symptom is subjective, and it is something that is experienced by the patient but cannot be seen or measured. If you tell the physician that you are dizzy or you are having knee pain or you are nauseated, you are giving the physician a symptom as he or she cannot see those complaints. It is very important for medical professionals to be able to discern between a sign and a symptom. Remember just alike a road sign can be seen, a complaint that someone has that can be seen or measured is a sign.

Eponyms are medical terms that carry the name of the person or place associated with the term. There are so many eponyms in the medical field. Every time someone discovers something new it seems that put his or her name on it. This is one of the reasons that the medical field is always evolving and changing, which requires us to stay up to date on terminology.

Alzheimer's disease—named after the German neurologist Alois Alzheimer—is a progressive mental deterioration.

Achilles tendon—the band of tissue that attaches the calf muscle to the heel bone. Achilles was a Greek hero during the Trojan War.

Notice the ending of eponyms -nym. Nym is a Greek term for name. We use acronyms frequently in the medical field. Acronyms are terms make from the initial letter of an abbreviation.

Abbreviations and symbols are short forms of terms used because they are easy to use and is more convenient. They are very common in the medical field. IM is the abbreviation for intramuscular. CABG means coronary artery bypass graft. IV means intravenous or pertaining to within the vein. Although abbreviations are commonly used, they can be dangerous for some. There are a few abbreviations that we use that can have more than one meaning dependent on the context in which they are used. Therefore, we must be very careful in using abbreviations and ensure that we understand our employers' rules and guidelines for using abbreviations. Most facilities have a do-not-use list that lets you know what abbreviations are not acceptable. The Joint Commission published a do-not-use list that has both abbreviations and symbols that should not be used.

Listening, speaking, reading, and writing are all tools that allow us to make medical terminology a great tool in which to communicate with physicians, colleagues, patients, and family.

What makes us a good listener? Is it eye contact, nodding our head, repeating what was said to us, or all of the above? All of the above. We must be able to listen to the people that are communicating with us for us to relay and document pertinent things that we heard.

No one likes to hear someone that cannot speak the language. Medical terminology is no different. It is one thing to be able to break that word down into its separate parts and quite another to be able to say the word with confidence. When we can speak the various words, it allow us to communicate with the medical world.

Remember when you were learning to read, everything looks foreign and did not make sense. However, with practice, you learned to read and form the words. Medical terminology might seem like a foreign language to you at this point; however, by the end of the text, you will have mastered the art of medical language. Our job as medical practitioners is made up of our ability to read and understand medical language. We then can take that information and communicate it as necessary.

Legibility is the last of the tools. Our writing must be legible. In other words, someone who we don't know may be looking at our writings and he or she must be able to accurately read it. While the medical profession has for the most part gone electronic, we must not completely rely on the computer to ensure that what we type is spelled correctly and written in the proper context. Proofreading out documentation will allow us to ensure that what we wrote not only made sense but was spelled correctly.

Therefore, now let's start decoding words. Remember all the way back to English class in high school, prefixes, suffixes, and vowels. This is going to be the foundation for the rest of the book. If you have a good understanding of how to break a word down to know what it means, medical terminology will come easy.

Most of the terms we will see are composed of a combining form and a suffix. The combining form is the subject of the term or what the term is about. It is comprised a root word and a combining vowel, which is usually an o. The suffix is the ending of the term. This tells us about the combining form. Is the term describing an anatomical feature, a procedure, a disease, a treatment, or something else?

In order to understand the word, we must be able to decode or break it down into simpler parts and then assign meanings to each part. Therefore, let's break down the word glossitis.

We want to check the word for its different parts:
Gloss/itis
Then, we need to assign meanings to the word parts:
Gloss/o—means tongue
Itis—means inflammation of

Therefore, based on our word parts, we have tongue inflammation of. Well that doesn't sound medically correct; therefore, we need to reverse the meaning of the suffix to the front of the translation. Therefore, for the word glossitis, we get inflammation of the tongue.

Combining Forms	Suffixes
Arthr/o	-algia
Gastr/o	-tomy
Ophthalm/o	-scope
Ot/o	-logy
Rhin/o	-plasty

Arthr/o = a joint
Gastr/o = the stomach (the organ)
Ophthalm/o = the eye
Ot/o = the ear
Rhin/o = the nose
-algia = pain
-tomy = an incision
-scope = an instrument to visually examine
-logy = the study of
-plasty = surgical repair

If we use the word rhinoplasty and break the word into its parts: rhin/o and plasty. We assign meaning to the word that is nose and surgical repair. Now we reverse the suffix to the beginning of the translation and we have surgical repair of the nose. Doesn't that sound more medically sound that nose job? Let's try one more before we move on to the five rules. The word is gastralgia. We need to assign meaning to the word parts. Gastr/a meaning stomach and algia meaning pain. Now we reverse the suffix to the beginning of the translation and we have pain in the stomach or pain of the stomach.

Utilizing what we know so far; The patient complained of chronic gastralgia. We know that this patient has pain in the stomach that is long term and returns.

There are five rules that we will discuss that are the foundation of decoding all medical terms.

Rule #1

If the suffix starts with a vowel, a combining vowel is not needed to join the parts.

Arthr/o + -itis = arthritis.

See how we did not need to keep the "o" because the suffix starts with a vowel.

Rule #2

If the suffix starts with a consonant, a combining vowel is needed to join the two word parts.

Arthr/o + -plasty = arthroplasty

Now the suffix starts with a consonant so we keep the combining vowel.

Rule #3

If a combining form ends with the same vowel that begins a suffix, one of the vowels is dropped.

Endocardi/o + -itis = endocarditis.

Now we have two potential vowels that would be together so we drop one of the vowels to create the word.

Rule #4

If two or more combining forms are used in a term, the combining vowel is retained between the two, regardless of whether the second combining form is a vowel or a suffix.

Gastr/o + enter/o + -itis = gastroenteritis

The "o" is dropped from enter/o when combined with a suffix because the suffix starts with a vowel. However, the "o" is kept between gastr/o and enter/o because they are two combining forms. The vowel/consonant issue only is important for suffixes.

Rule #5

Sometimes when two or more combining forms are used to make a term, special notice needs to be paid to the order in which the combining forms are joined.

Esophagi/o + gastr/o + duoden/o + -scopy = esophagogastroduodenoscopy

The normal route of the digestive system is from the esophagus (esophag/o) to the stomach (gastr/o) to the first part of the small intestine, the duodenum (duoden/o).

Now it is time to start building the word bank. Let's start with noun suffixes. A noun is a person place or thing.

Structure, thing

-is (ex: hypodermis)

Structure, thing, membrane

-um (ex: endocardium)

Small, tiny

-icle, -ole, -ule (ex: cuticle, arteriole, and venule)

Hypodermis is the structure under the skin.

Endocardium is the membrane within the heart.

Cuticle is the little skin around your nail. Arteriole is a little artery, and venule is a little vein.

Adjective suffixes describe something. The adjective that means pertaining to are the following:

-ac	cardiac
-al	cervical
-ar	valvular
-ary	coronary
-eal	esophageal
-ic	hypodermic
-ous	subcutaneous

Therefore, cardiac is pertaining to the heart. We don't know what exactly, but we know it's pertaining to the heart.

Digital is pertaining to a finger or toe.
Vavular is pertaining to a valve.
Mammary is pertaining to the breast.
Hypodermic is pertaining to below the skin.
Subcutaneous is also pertaining to below the skin.

Pathology Suffixes	
-algia	cephalalgia
-emia	hyperlipidemia
-ia	agastria
-itis	tonsillitis

Cephal/o means head, and -algia is yet a suffix for pain. Therefore, this term describes pain in the head, or a headache.

Hyperlipidemia is a blood condition of excessive fats.
Agastria is a condition of no stomach.
Tonsillitis is inflammation of the tonsils.

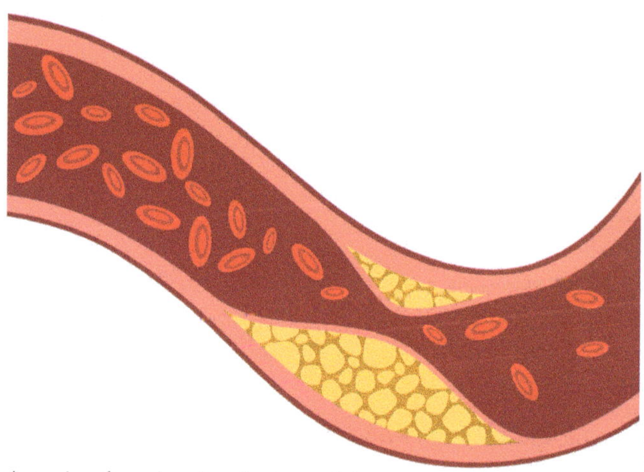

Arteriosclerosis—hardening of the arteries

Diagnostic Suffixes	
-graphy	mammography
-metry	spirometry
-opsy	biopsy
-scopy	hysteroscopy

Mammography is the process of recording the breasts.
Spirometry is the process of measurement of breathing.
Biopsy is the process of viewing living tissue.
Hysteroscopy is a process of viewing the uterus.

Therapeutic Suffixes	
-ectomy	gastrectomy
-plasty	rhinoplasty
-stomy	colostomy
-tomy	osteotomy
-tripsy	lithotripsy

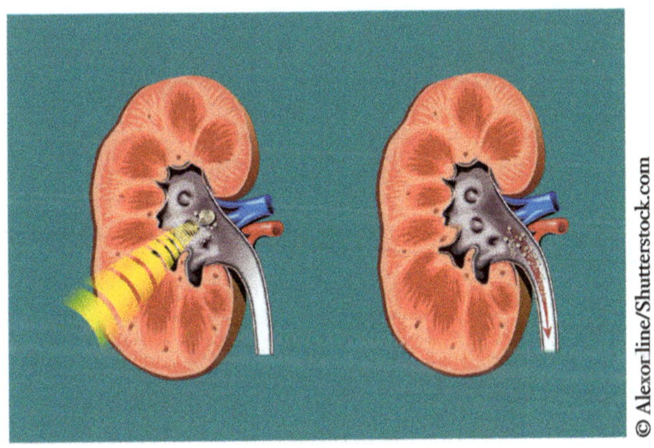

Lithotripsy

Gastrectomy is a removal or resection (they mean the same) of the stomach.

Rhinoplasty is a surgical repair of the nose. Sometimes this also means a cosmetic repair of the nose—something that insurance rarely covers.

A colostomy is a new opening of the large intestine.

Osteotomy is an incision of bone.

Lithotripsy is a crushing of a stone.

Instrument Suffixes	
-graph	electrocardiograph
-meter	thermometer
-scope	ophthalmoscope

An electrocardiograph is an instrument to record the electrical activity of the heart. The record that it makes is an electrocardiogram. You may have seen the abbreviation, ECG or EKG.

A thermometer is an instrument to measure heat or temperature.

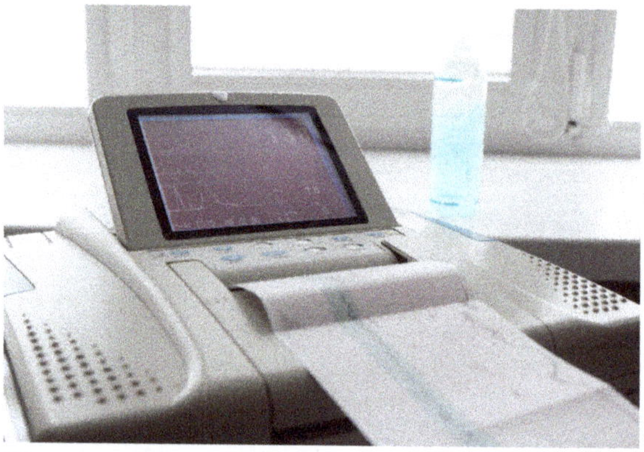
© Eight Photo/Shutterstock.com

Electrocardiograph

An ophthalmoscope is an instrument to view the eye.

Prefixes are attached directly to the beginning of the term and they may have more than one meaning. Examples of prefixes are: a-, an-, ante-, and anti-.

a-	apneic
an-	anophthalmia
ante-	anteversion
anti-	antibacterial

Pertaining to not breathing is the definition for the term "apneic." As in many definitions, this does not give you the entire story. Apnea (the noun) is a condition of temporary lack of breathing.

Anophthalmia means a condition of no eye.

Anteversion is the process of turning forward.

Antibacterial is pertaining to against bacteria (like the wipes you may use to clean).

dys-	dystrophy
endo-, end-	endoscopy
epi-	epigastric

Dystrophy is a condition of abnormal nourishment.

Endoscopy is the process of viewing within.

Epigastric means pertaining to above the stomach.

hyper-	hyperglycemia
hypo-	hypoglossal
inter-	intervertebral
intra-	intradermal

para-, par-	paraphilia
per-	percutaneous
peri-	pericardium
pre-	prenatal
poly-	polyneuritis
post-	postictal
sub-	subhepatic

These two prefixes are very common, but look very similar.
Hyperglycemia is a blood condition of excessive sugar.
Hypoglossal is pertaining to below the tongue.
Intervertebral means pertaining to between two backbones.
Intradermal means pertaining to within the skin.
Para- and par- mean abnormal (or sometimes near).
Paraphilia is an abnormal attraction to something. An example is pedophilia, which would be an attraction to what? (children)
Percutaneous means pertaining to through the skin.
Pericardium is the membrane surrounding the heart.
Prenatal means pertaining to before birth.
Polyneuritis is an inflammation of many nerves. Remember polysomnographer?
Postictal is pertaining to after a seizure.
Subhepatic is pertaining to below the liver.

Singular and Plural Endings	
Singular:	**Plural:**
Vertebra	vertebrae
Arthrosis	arthroses
Appendix	appendices
Arthritis	arthritides
Phalanx	phalanges
Endocardium	endocardia
Digitus	digiti
Therapy	therapies

These singular/plural endings are the result of the Greek and Latin origins of our terminology.

For the singulars, if the term ends in the bolded letter/s, drop them and add the bolded letter/s in the plural column.

A vertebra is a backbone.

Arthrosis is an abnormal condition of a joint.

Appendix usually refers to an addition as in the vermiform appendix that hangs off of the first part of the large intestine.

A phalanx is a bone in a finger or toe.

The endocardium is the membrane that lines the heart.

A digitus is a finger or toe.

A therapy is another name for treatment.

There always has to be unusual letter combinations and medical terminology is not different. Below are a few examples of how these unusual letter combinations are used and pronounced.

eu	euthyroid
ph	phalanx
pn	pneumonitis
ps	psychology
pt	ptosis
rh, rrh	rhinitis
x	xeroderma

Many of these terms just plain look weird. However, you need to be able to pronounce them. Your text will give you a pronunciation for each one, but be aware of some general rules.

eu has a sound like the word "you." Euthyroid means a good, normal thyroid gland.
ph has an "f" sound. Again, a phalanx is a finger or toe bone.
pn has an "n" sound. Pneumonitis is an inflammation of the lungs.
ps has an "s" sound. Psychology is the study of the mind.
pt has a "t" sound. Ptosis is a drooping or sagging.
rh, rrh have an "r" sound. Rhinitis is an inflammation of the nose.
x has a "z" sound. Xeroderma is a condition of dry skin. (Think Xerox, which got its name from its use of a dry ink.)

Medical terminology is a learned art. Yes, there is a lot of memorization required to understand what we are trying to get across to someone, but if we gain a good foundation of understanding prefixes, suffixes, and root words, we will be well our way to mastery. Beginning in Chapter 3, we will separate the majority of terms into four categories.

Anatomy and physiology
Pathology (disease and disorders)
Diagnostic procedures (tests)
Therapeutic interventions (treatments)

CHAPTER 2

Structure of the Body and Directional Terms

In order for the body to function properly, it is constantly trying to maintain balance within the body. This process is known as homeostasis. Home/o means same and -statis means controlling. Our body attempts to get back to homeostasis or the body's happy place. The body either expends or conserves energy. Our body is in constant regulation mode and anything we do (eat, drink, exercise, or sleep) and everything that we eat or drink. Age, gender, and weight also play an important role in our body's ability to maintain homeostasis.

Homeostasis (home/o + -stasis)
- Energy conversion
  - Metabolism (meta-)
  - Anabolism (ana-)
  - Catabolism (cata-)

Homeostasis: home/o means same and -stasis means controlling. Homeostasis is a normal process of maintaining balance within the body.

Anabolism is the building up [or literally, a process of throwing up (as in building up)], while catabolism is the process of throwing down (as in breaking down). Metabolism is the total process of building up and breaking down the body's energy stores.

In order to live, cells need a constant supply of energy.

The prefix meta- means "change" (although we will see this term with another meaning later). Bol/o means to throw or throwing. The suffix -ism means the state of. Metabolism is the process of continually building up and breaking down of substances that provide energy. The ancient Greeks thought of it as substances being changed by the process of throwing.

Tissues (hist/o)
- Parenchymal vs. stromal
- Four types of tissues
  - Epithelial
  - Connective
  - Muscular
  - Nervous

Parenchymal (does the work of an organ) and stromal (is supportive in nature) tissues (the kidneys are parenchymal, and the ureters are stromal).

Tissue types:

Epithelial tissue acts as an internal or external covering for organs most prone to cancer because of contact with the environment.
Connective tissue has the property of an internal structural network.
Muscular tissue has the unique ability to contract and relax.
Nervous tissue serves to provide for the transmission of information within the body.

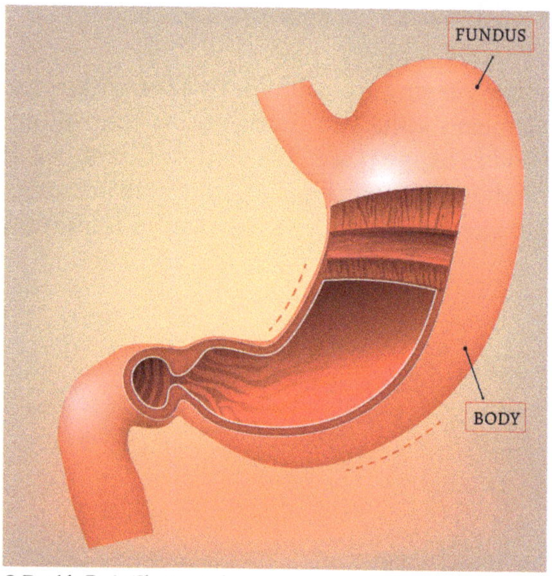

© Double Brain/Shutterstock.com

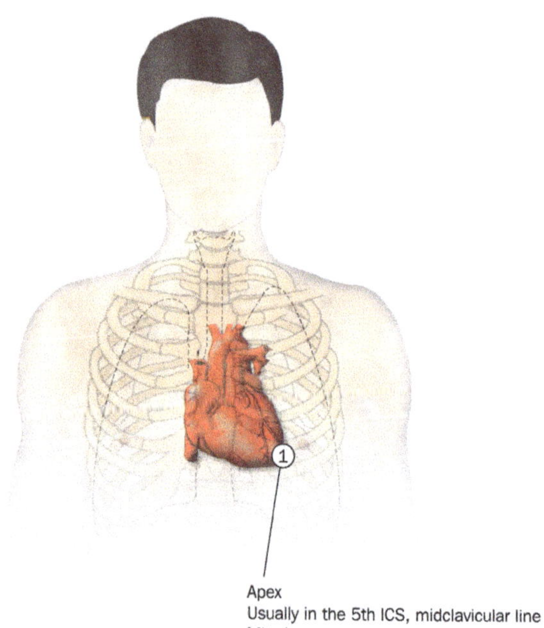

© Blamb/Shutterstock.com

Epithelial tissues include the outer layer of the skin or lining of the digestive tract. Connective tissue includes bone, blood, and fat. Muscular tissue includes heart, skeletal, and visceral muscles, and nervous tissue includes the nerves, spinal cord, and brain.

Organs (organ/o, viscer/o) are found throughout or body. We will discuss specific organs within each chapter but it is important to understand that organs can be instrumental in more than one body system. Within organs, we can have an arrangement of various types of tissues. Take the heart as an example. The heart has epithelial tissue, which is the endocardium (the lining of the chambers of the heart). The heart also has muscular tissue or myocardium (the muscle of the heart).

Not only do we need to know the names of organs, we need to know the locations of organs. There is very specific terminology that is used to describe specific locations.

The apex is the pointed extremity of an organ. In the heart, this is at the bottom, whereas in the lungs, the apex is at the top. The plural of apex is apices. (Remember the rule? If a term ends in -ex, it can be made plural by dropping the ex and adding ices.)

The body of an organ is the largest or the most important part of an organ. A synonym is corpus. Note that the combining forms are corpor/o, som/o, and somat/o. The diagram here is of the stomach with the body noted.

The fundus is the base or the deepest part of an organ. Here we have the uterine fundus illustrated. Fundal height is an important measurement when determining the age of the fetus. It is measured from the pubic bone to the top of the uterus.

The anatomical position is the frame of reference that is used to describe the surface anatomy. In order to be in the anatomical position, a person is standing erect, face forward, arms at sides with palms facing forward, and toes pointed forward. This is the point of reference that is most frequently used when comparing the location of one structure in relation to another structure.

The ventral surface of the body refer to the front of the body when someone is in the anatomical position. There are several points of reference and prefixes that need to be addressed:

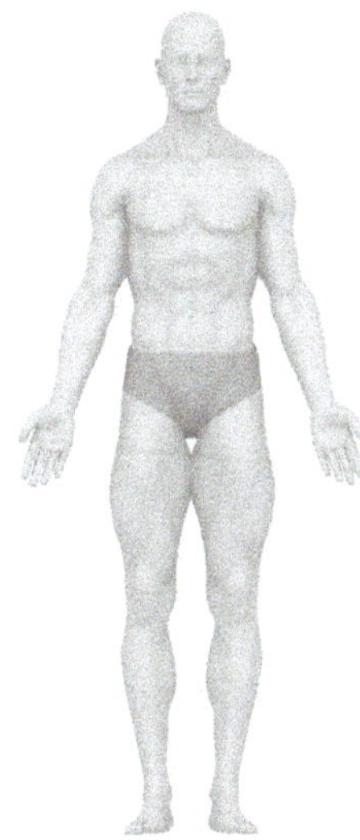

Anatomical Position

Ventral Surface Anatomy—Head and Neck

Buccal means pertaining to the cheek. Bucc/o is a combining form for the cheek.

Cephalic means pertaining to the head. Cephal/o means the head.

Cervical means pertaining to the neck. Cervic/o means the neck. **Be careful! In the female reproductive system, cervic/o refers to the neck of the cervix. Pay attention to the context of what you are reading to understand which "neck" is being talked about.**

Cranial means pertaining to the skull. Crani/o means the skull.

Facial means pertaining to the face. Faci/o means the face. Another Be Careful! Don't confuse faci/o with fasci/o, the tough outer covering of the muscles.

Frontal literally means pertaining to the front. In the context of surface anatomy, it refers to the forehead.

Mental means pertaining to the chin when you are talking about surface anatomy of the face. The mental foramina are small holes in the bone of the lower jaw that provide an entrance/exit for blood vessels and nerves.

Nasal means pertaining to the nose. Nas/o is a combining form for the nose.

Ocular means pertaining to the eye. Ocul/o is a combining form for the eye.

Oral means pertaining the mouth. Or/o is a combining form for the mouth.

Otic means pertaining to the ear. Ot/o is a combining form for the ear.

In this section, you will notice that cervical has two meanings. Cervic/o means neck. Cervical means pertaining to the neck. That can be the neck that our head is attached to or in a female the neck of the cervix. Be very careful and make sure that the context in which the term is used is correct. This is an easy mistake to make if we are not aware of the multiple meanings.

Ventral Surface Anatomy—Truck

Abdominal means pertaining to the abdomen. Abdomin/o is one of the combining forms for the abdomen. Don't confuse the abdomen with the stomach. The abdomen is a region, not an organ.

Axillary means pertaining to the armpit. Axill/o is the combining form for the armpit.

Coxal means pertaining to the hip. Cox/o is a combining form for the hip.

Deltoid means resembling a triangle, which describes the muscle that covers the shoulder. Delt/o is the combining form for the deltoid muscle.

Inguinal means pertaining to in the groin. Inguin/o is a combining form for the groin.

Mammary means pertaining to the breast. Mamm/o is a combining form for the breast.

Pelvic means pertaining to the pelvis. The combining form for pelvis is pelv/i.

Sternal means pertaining to the sternum (the breastbone). Stern/o is a combining form for the sternum.

Thoracic means pertaining to the chest. Thorac/o is a combining form for the chest.

Umbilical means pertaining to the navel (belly button). Umbilic/o is a combining form for the umbilicus.

Ventral Surface Anatomy—Arms

Antecubital means pertaining to the front (ante-) of the elbow (cubit/o).

Brachial means pertaining to the arm. Brachi/o is a combining form for the arm.

Carpal means pertaining to the wrist. Carp/o is a combining form for the wrist.

Manual is a combining form for the hand. Man/u is a combining form for the hand.

Palmar means pertaining to the palm of the hand. Palm/o is a combining form for the palm.

Digital means pertaining to a whole finger or toe. Digit/o is a combining form for the finger or toe.

Ventral Surface Anatomy—Legs

Crural means pertaining to the leg. Crur/o is a combining form for the leg.

Femoral means pertaining to the thigh. The femur is the thighbone. Femor/o means the thighbone.

Patellar means pertaining to the knee. Patell/a is a combining form for the knee and kneecap.

Pedal means pertaining to the foot. Ped/o is a combining form for the foot. However, Be Careful! Don't confuse ped//o meaning foot with ped/o meaning children. Context rules!

Plantar means pertaining to the sole of the foot. Plant/o is a combining form for the sole.

Tarsal means pertaining to the ankle. Tars/o is a combining form for the ankle and the tarsals (ankle bones).

The dorsal surface anatomy is looking at the body from the back. You may recognize the word dorsal and relate it to the dorsal fin of a dolphin. This fin is on the dolphins back or dorsal surface. There are not as many terms or structures on the dorsal side of the body.

Dorsal Surface Anatomy

Acromial means pertaining to the shoulder. Acromi/o is a combining form for the shoulder or the acromion process. It refers to the highest point of the shoulder.

Dorsal means pertaining to the back. Dors/o is a combining form for the back.

Gluteal means pertaining to the buttocks. Glute/o is a combining form for the buttocks.

Lumbar means pertaining to the loins, or the lower back. Llumb/o means lower back or loins.

Nuchal means pertaining to the neck. Nuch/o means neck.

Perineal means pertaining to the perineum.

Sacral means pertaining to the sacrum. As you can see, the sacrum is below the lumbar region. Sacr/o means the sacrum. Be careful here. Sarc/o looks very similar but means flesh.

Scapular means pertaining to the scapula (shoulder blade).

Vertebral means pertaining to the vertebrae, the bones in the back. Vertebr/o means the vertebrae.

Olecranal means pertaining to the elbow. Olecran/o is a combining form for the elbow.

Popliteal means pertaining to the back of the knee. Poplite/o is a combining form for the back of the knee.

Sural means pertaining to the calf. Sur/o is a combining form for the calf.

We have reviewed the ventral and dorsal surfaces, and we need to look at positional and directional terms. Again, when referring to positional and directional terms, remember the anatomical position as these terms are based on someone standing in the anatomical position.

- Anterior (anter/o)
  - ant
  - Ventral (ventr/o)
- Posterior (poster/o)
  - pos
  - Dorsal (dors/o)

Anterior means pertaining to the front. It's abbreviated *ant* and has a synonym, ventral. Ventr/o, the combining form used in ventral, means the "belly side," which you can understand to mean the same as the front.

The back is posterior with an abbreviation of *pos*. The synonym for posterior is dorsal.

Ventral and dorsal are also used to describe the back and the belly side of animals. (It's kind of hard to determine if the area under a dog or cat's face is part of its back or front. If you think of having the animal stand on its back feet, you can easily see that it's part of the belly side, or the ventral surface.)

Let's put some of these words to work and utilize them in the real world.

Anteroposterior and posteroanterior:

Anteroposterior means from front to back. It is abbreviated AP.

Posteroanterior means from back to front. It is abbreviated PA.

Can you see how it is describing the direction of the x-ray beam? The direction that the beam will travel will determine whether it is an AP or PA x-ray.

- Superior (super/o)
  - sup
  - Cephalad (cephal/o)
- Inferior (infer/o)
  - inf
  - Caudad (caud/o)

Superior means pertaining to upward. Super/o is a combining form meaning upward. The abbreviation for superior is sup. Cepahlad means toward the head. Cephal/o is a combining form meaning the head. The suffix *-ad* means "toward."

Inferior means pertaining to downward. Infer/o is a combining form meaning downward. Inf is the combining form. Caudad means toward the tail. Caud/o is the combining form for the tail.

- ☐ Medial (medi/o)
- ☐ Lateral (later/o)
  Lat

Medial means pertaining to the middle (doesn't it look like that?) with medi/o being a combining form for middle.

Lateral means pertaining to the side. Later/o is a combining form for the side. The abbreviation is lat.

- ☐ Ipsilateral (ipsi-)
- ☐ Contralateral (contra-)

Ipsilateral means pertaining to the same side. The prefix ipsi- means the same.

Contralateral means pertaining to the opposite side. Contra- is a prefix meaning the opposite.

- ☐ Unilateral (uni-)
- ☐ Bilateral (bi-)

Unilateral means pertaining to one side. Uni- is a prefix for one.

Bilateral means pertaining to two sides. Bi- is a prefix meaning two. Don't confuse the prefix bi- with the combining form bi/o meaning life, living.

- ☐ Proximal (proxim/o)
- ☐ Distal (dist/o)

Proximal means pertaining to near the point of origin. Proxim/o is a combining form for near.

Distal means pertaining to farther from the point of origin. Dist/o is a combining form for far.

A frame of reference is important in this definition. That's why the definition includes "the point of origin." If the terms are used to describe a location that is nearer to or farther from the points of origin of the arms and legs, it's referring to the shoulders and hips, respectively.

If proximal and distal are used to describe sites within the body, it is referring to the beginning and end of the organ.

Hold out your arm and say, "the wrist is ________ to the elbow." The wrist is distal to the elbow because it is farther from the shoulder (the point of attachment) than the elbow is. But! The elbow is ______ to the wrist. The elbow is proximal to the wrist because it is closer to the shoulder than the wrist.

Superficial means pertaining to the surface. A superficial wound is on the surface. External is used to mean the same as superficial.
Deep means away from the surface of the body. This means the same as internal.

When describing how a person is lying, we use supine and prone. These are much better descriptive terms than found them on their back or stomach. Again utilizing the medically correct term will not only allow us to speak medical language but also allow us to use the terms that are generally accepted in the medical field.

A patient who is in the supine position is lying on his or her back.
A patient who is in the prone position is lying on his or her stomach.

- Dextrad (dextr/o)
- Sinistrad (sinistr/o, levo-)

Dextrad means toward the right, while sinistrad means toward the left. Note that there is one combining form for the right (dextr/o), while the left has a combining form (sinistr/o) and a prefix (levo-).

- Afferent (af-)
- Efferent (ef-)

Afferent means pertaining to carrying (fer/o) toward (af-) a structure.
Efferent means pertaining to carrying (fer/o) away from (ef-) a structure.
You can see how afferent vessels carry substances toward a structure, like the kidney, while efferent vessels carry substances away from the structure.

- Dorsal cavities
  - Cranial (crani/o)
  - Spinal (spin/o)
- Ventral cavities
  - Thoracic (thorac/o)
  - Abdominal (abdomin/o)
  - Pelvic (pelv/i)

The body is composed of cavities in the back of the body, the dorsal cavities, and in the front of the body, the ventral cavities.

The dorsal cavities are the cranial cavity (remember that crani/o means skull?) and the spinal cavity. Spin/o is a combining form for the spine.

The ventral cavities are the thoracic cavity (thorac/o means chest), the abdominal cavity (abdomin/o means abdomen), and the pelvic cavity (pelv/i is a combining form for the pelvis).

- Ventral cavity
  - Thoracic
    - Mediastinum (mediastin/o)
    - Pleural cavity (pleur/o)
  - Abdominal
    - Diaphragm (diaphragm/o, diaphragmat/o, or phren/o)
    - Peritoneum (peritone/o)
  - Pelvic

The thoracic cavity is filled with the lungs, the heart, the esophagus, and the trachea (windpipe). It too has cavities. The space between the lungs is called the mediastinum (combining form is mediastin/o). The double-folded membrane that surrounds the lungs is termed the pleura. The space between the folds is called the pleural cavity.

The abdominal cavity contains the stomach, liver, and intestines (these are the major structures). It is separated from the thoracic cavity by a muscle called the diaphragm (combining forms are diaphragm/o, diaphragmat/o, and phren/o). The cavity is lined with a highly vascular (lots of vessels) membrane called the peritoneum (combining form is peritone/o).

The pelvic cavity, although often listed with the abdominal cavity, contains the bladder and reproductive organs.

If the abdominal and pelvic cavities are referred to together, the cavity is the abdominopelvic cavity.

The abdominopelvic quadrants (sections) are how we divide the abdomen into sections. You will see this region divided into either four or nine quadrants. For the purpose of this text, we will divide the abdomen into four quadrants. It is imperative that we understand where certain organs and structures are in each of these quadrants.

- Right upper quadrant (RUQ)
  - Liver
- Left upper quadrant (LUQ)
  - Stomach and spleen
- Right lower quadrant (RLQ)
  - Appendix and McBurney's point
- Left lower quadrant (LLQ)
  - Munro's point

Abdominopelvic quadrants divide the area into four segments (quadri- means four). They are either upper or lower and left or right.

The right upper quadrant is the location of the liver, while the left upper quadrant is the location of the stomach and spleen.

The right lower quadrant is the location of the appendix, intestines, and ovaries in the female. The location directly above the appendix (approximately two-thirds of the way between the hipbone and the navel) is called McBurney's point. The left lower quadrant contains the same organs as the right, excepting the appendix. Munro's point, a location about halfway between the hipbone and navel in this quadrant, is the standard site of entrance for abdominal laparoscopic surgery.

Within the medical field, you will see these quadrants referred to as: *RUQ, LUQ, RLQ, and LLQ.*

For myself, the most challenging part of medical terminology was learning and understanding the planes of the body. Some of the following terms are fairly straightforward, while some are more challenging. We will try and break these down so they are easily understood.

- Sagittal
  - Midsagittal

Planes are slices of the body that are used in imaging.

Sagittal separates the sides; the right from the left. Midsagittal separates them exactly in the middle. This plane essentially cuts the body in half. Remember we are looking at the body in its anatomical position.

- Frontal/coronal

Frontal/coronal separates the front from the back into anterior and posterior portions.

- Transverse

Transverse planes separate the body into superior and inferior portions.

Oblique planes, not as commonly used, divide the body at a slanted angle. These are very common planes used when someone has a CT scan.

You have made it through all of the terms that give you a good foundation to begin exploring the different body systems. In the coming chapters, we will break down each body system and employ the definitions and terms in the first two chapters to learn to break down the terms in each system; therefore, we can understand what these terms mean.

CHAPTER 3

Integumentary

The integumentary system is made up of the skin, hair, nails, sebaceous glands, and the sweat glands. The skin is the external covering of the body and is the largest organ of the body. In an average adult, the skin weighs more than 6 pounds and covers roughly 3,000 square inches. The skins has four main functions: protection, regulation, sensation, and secretion.

The skins has many functions and serve a very important purpose in our ability to function. The skin is the first line of defense (protection) that the body uses to fight bacteria and other harmful organisms that try to get into the deeper tissues. If the skin is broken, the line of defense is breached and bacteria or other harmful agents have direct access to the body. The skin also helps to inhibit the loss of fluids and electrolytes; but the skin also repels water. The skin also protects us against too much exposure to UV rays and it helps to produce the body's supply of vitamin D.

- The sensation perceived by the skin is the sense of touch. Receptors in the skin allow an individual to know when he or she is in contact with the environment. These are the terms that relate to an excessive sensation of touch (hyperesthesia) and a lack of sensation of feeling (anesthesia).
- Vitamin D, a substance important to normal development of teeth and bones, is synthesized by the skin.
- Dermatology is the study of the skin. Dermat/o = skin + -logy = study of the skin. A dermatologist is one who specializes in the study of the skin. Dermat/o = skin + -logist = one who specializes in the study of the skin.

Our skins also help us in our ability to regulate our temperature. When it is cold, our body shivers in an attempt to generate heat. When it is hot, our body sweats in an attempt to cool down the body.

The combining forms for the skin are derm/o, dermat/o, cutane/o, and cut/o. Some of them might sounds familiar.

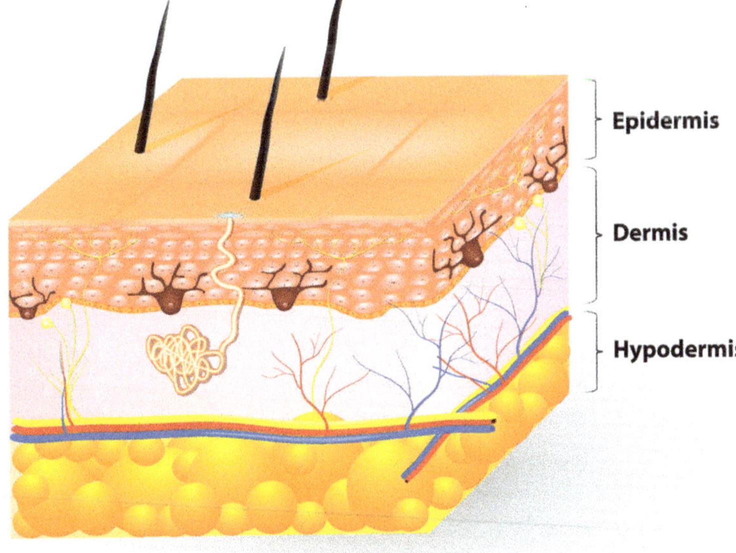

© Designua/Shutterstock.com

The skin is arranged in layers. The top layer is the epidermis (epi- meaning above, or upon, derm/o for skin, and -is for structure). Hence, the epidermis is the top layer of the skin. The deepest layer of the epidermis is the site of continual new growth for skin cells along with the production of the substance melanin, which gives the skin its color. Pigmentation is governed by the melanocytes (melan/o = black + -cyte = cell) that produce a dark pigment called melanin. In the presence of sunlight, the melanocytes increase their production of melanin, providing a form of protection against ultraviolet light.

The dermis (also called the corium) is the true layer of the skin; it holds the blood vessels, oil and sweat glands, and nerves for sensation.

- Structures
  - Blood and lymphatic vessels
  - Nerves
  - Hair follicles (follicul/o)
  - Sebaceous (sebac/o) and sudoriferous glands (sudor/i)

Underneath the dermis is the layer called the hypodermis or subcutaneous (hypo- under or beneath, derm/o again for skin, and -is for structure). Sub- means under or below, cutane/o means skin, and -ous means pertaining to. Therefore, the two names both refer to the structure under the skin. This tissue is filled with fat (adip/o). Everyone has a layer of adipose tissue that helps to insulate and cushion the body.

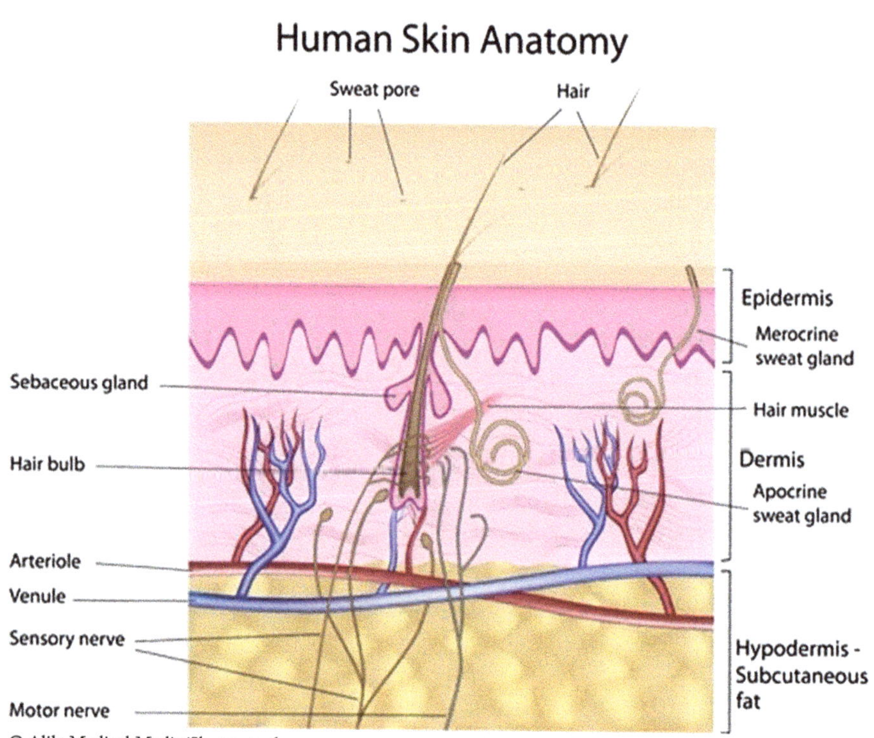

There are two glands in the skin that produce sweat and oil. The sudoriferous (sweat) glands and the sebaceous (oil) glands.

The sudoriferous glands (sudor/i = sweat + -ferous = pertaining to carrying), also called the sweat glands, are instrumental in the regulation of body temperature. Note that the combining form for the sweat glands is hidraden/o, a composite of hidr/o for sweat and aden/o for gland. You may see the term "sudor" used to mean sweat, but it is used rarely.

Perspiration is a much more common term, and it occurs through tiny openings in the skin called pores. These pores are present on the soles of the feet, the palms of the hands, the axillae (axill/o = armpit), the upper lip, and the forehead.

Sebaceous glands secrete an oily substance termed "sebum," which serves to lubricate the hair and the skin. Note that the combining form is not tricky, it's simply seb/o.

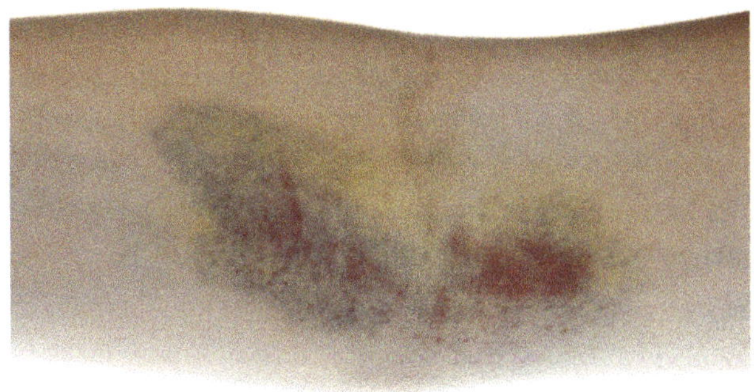

An example of hematoma

The combining forms for the hair are trich/o (pronounced trick) and pil/o. The root of each strand of hair is in the dermis, and it, along with its covering, is referred to as the hair follicle (combining form follicul/o). The part of the hair that you can see is called the shaft, and underneath the shaft is the nipple-shaped structure called the papilla. You'll find that the combining form for the papilla (papill/o) is used throughout terminology (in the terms for the eye and, obviously, in the female

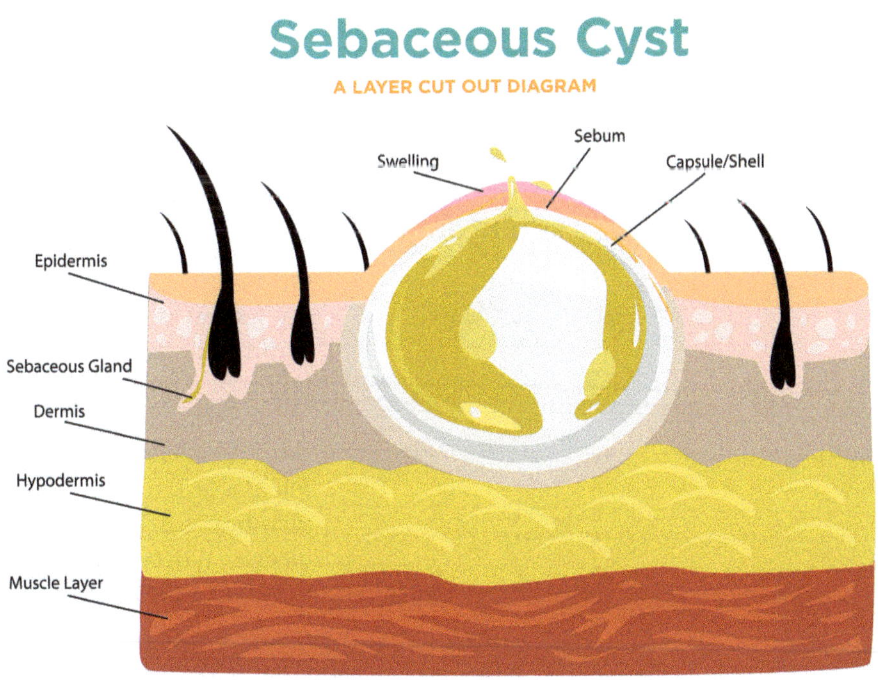

reproductive system, too). The cells on the top of the papilla are responsible for the formation of hair. When these cells die, for whatever reason, hair loss occurs.

There are also two kinds of lesions, a localized abnormality of the skin. There are primary and secondary lesions. Primary skin lesions are the ones that initially occur as the result of trauma or disease. Secondary lesions are those that have evolved from their primary forms. There are different types of primary lesions; nodules, cysts, tumors, and hematomas. Nodules are palpable solid lesions. Cysts are nodules that are filled with a semisolid material, like a keratinous cyst (also called a sebaceous cyst). Tumors are nodules that are larger than 2 cm (slightly less than an inch). The term "tumor" can be used to explain any mass or swelling, including neoplasms.

Hematomas are collections of extravasated (leaked) blood that are trapped in the tissues and can be felt by the examiner.

Ecchymosis (bruise) is a hemorrhage or extravasation of blood into the subcutaneous tissue. It is nonpalpable, but generally darkens the skin.

A petechia is a tiny ecchymosis in the dermal layer.

Purpura is a massive hemorrhage into the tissues under the skin.

All of these terms are forms of extravasation, which means the process of a substance (blood or lymph) leaking outside of a vessel into surrounding tissues.

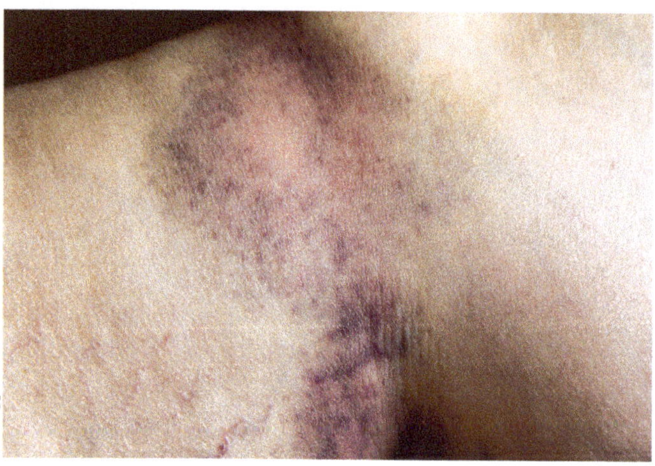

Ecchymosis

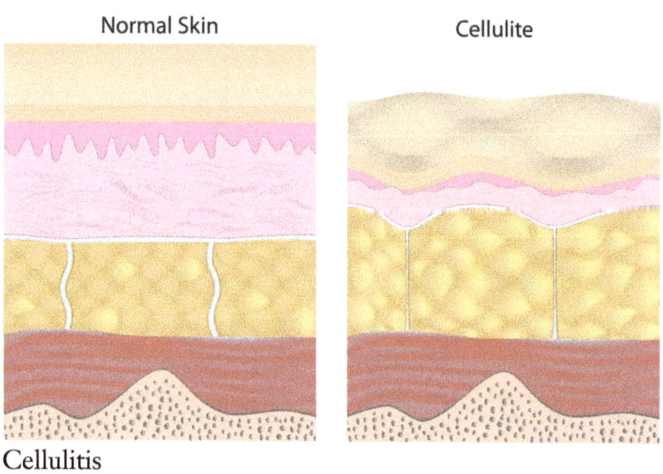

Cellulitis

A vesicle is a circumscribed elevated lesion that is filled with fluid and smaller than ½ cm. If it's larger than ½ cm, it is termed a bulla. We also refer to this as a blister.

A pustule is like a vesicle, but it is a raised lesion that is filled with pus as the result of an infection.

If skin is atrophied, it is characterized as being paper thin, wasted skin. An example is the thinning skin of the elderly or stretch marks that result from rapid weight gain.

A cicatrix is a scar, while a keloid is an overgrowth of tissue at the site of an injury.

Eschar is dried serum, blood, and/or pus that can occur at the site of an injury or a burn.

A fissure is a crack-like lesion of the skin. An ulcer is a circumscribed crater-like lesion of the skin or a mucous membrane. It's important to note that ulcers can occur on the outer surface of the body as well on the inside.

Atopic dermatitis is a chronic, pruritic superficial inflammation of the skin that usually occurs in families that have a history of allergic disorders. Cellulitis is a bacterial inflammation that is diffuse, spreading, and occurs within solid tissues.

Contact dermatitis is an inflammation of the skin that occurs as an irritated or allergic response. Eczema is a superficial inflammation of the skin characterized by vesicles, lesions that "weep," and pruritus. It is also referred to as dermatitis.

Folliculitis is an inflammation of the hair follicles (follicul/o=follicle). These inflammations can be superficial or deep, acute or chronic.

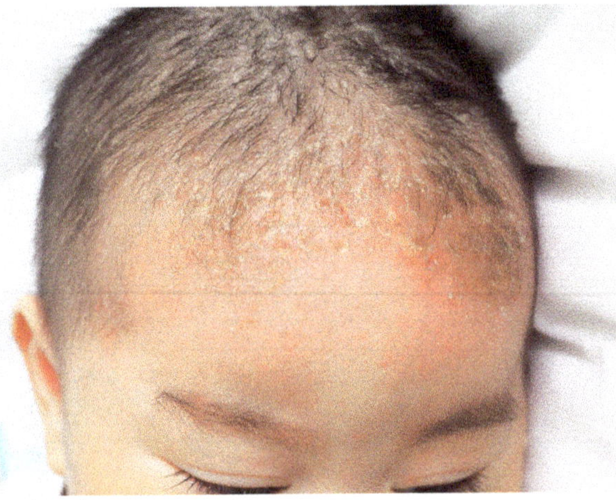
Seborrheic Dermatitis

Seborrheic dermatitis is an inflammatory scaly disease of the face and scalp. This is very common in children and is referred to as cradle cap. A furuncle is a localized staph infection that begins in a gland or hair follicle and is red, swollen, and painful. Impetigo is a superficial vesiculopustular skin infection that usually affects children. It can also be highly contagious.

Candidiasis is a yeast infection that is also called moniliasis.

Fungal infections of the skin are also termed dermatomycosis. Dermat/o = skin, myc/o = fungus, and -osis = abnormal condition. Naming the fungal infections by the specific body area is accomplished by using the term *tinea* for fungus and a second term indicating the area of the body. Tinea capitis is a fungal infection of the head (capit/o = head), tinea corporis of the body (corpor/o = body), tinea cruris (crur/o = leg) of the groin (commonly called "jock itch"), and tinea pedis of the foot (ped/o = foot) (known as athlete's foot).

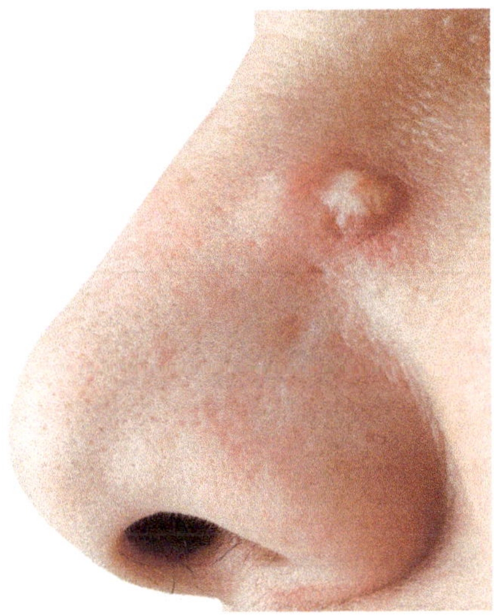
Furuncle

There are two parasitic infestations that are very common are lice and mites. Pediculosis is an infestation with lice, while scabies is an infestation with mites. Infestation with scabies causes an itchy (pruritic) papular rash.

Viral infections are very different than bacterial infections. Herpes simplex virus ranges from

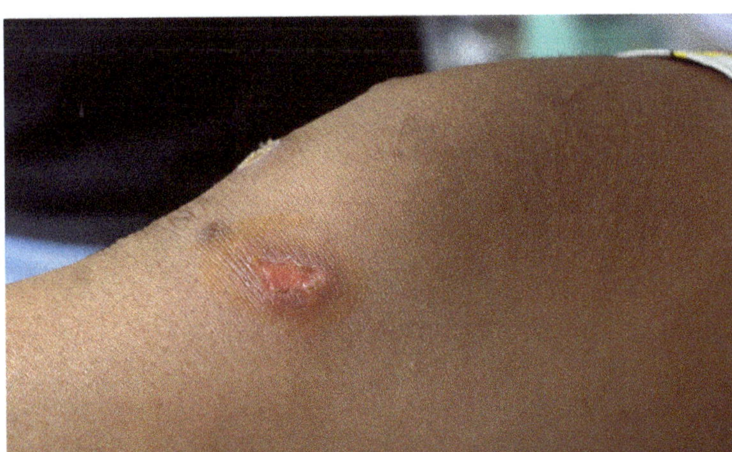
Impetigo

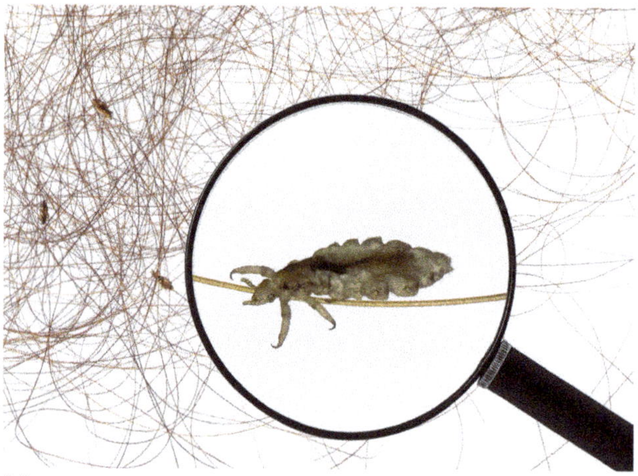

Lice

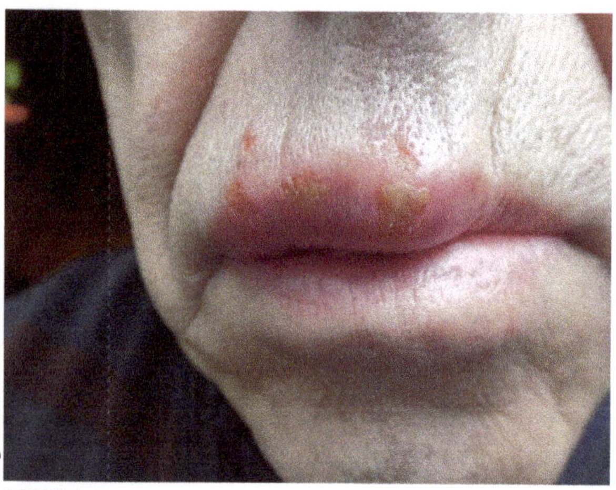

HSV-1

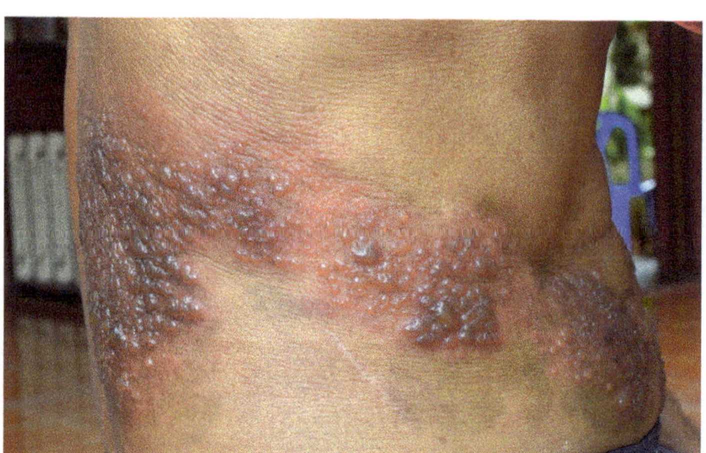

Herpes Zoster

fever blisters to shingles. The herpes virus comes in several forms and one of those forms is the sexually transmitted disease.

Exanthematous diseases are those that are characterized by a rash (exanthem). Measles, mumps, fifth disease, rubeola, and chicken pox are examples of exanthematous diseases.

Herpes simplex virus (HSV): These viral infections cause clusters of small vesicles on raised inflammatory sites on the skin or mucosa.

HSV-1 causes fever blisters/cold sores/herpetic stomatitis (they're all synonyms for each other) and keratitis, an inflammation of the cornea. Point out that the cornea is the hard outer covering of the eye. It uses the same combining forms (corne/o and kerat/o) as the combining forms used to describe hard, horny conditions of the skin. Remember that stomat/o means mouth, not stomach.

HSV-2 is more commonly known as genital herpes.

Herpes zoster is an acute painful rash caused by a reactivation of the latent varicella zoster virus (the one that causes chicken pox). This disorder is more commonly referred to as shingles.

Verruca is a medical term for a wart. It is caused by a virus and can appear on the skin in various locations on the body. For example, plantar warts appear on the sole of the foot (the plantar surface). Note the plural form of the term *verruca* (verrucae).

Acne vulgaris (vulgaris means common) is an inflammatory disease of the sebaceous glands. The lesions are papules, pustules, inflamed nodules, and comedones (s. comedo). A comedo is a plug of sebum that partially blocks a pore. Open comedones are blackheads, while closed comedones are whiteheads.

Alopecia is the term for hair loss or baldness. Hair loss occurs for a number of reasons including aging, disease, or genetic factors. Alopecia comes from the Greek term *alopekia*, meaning fox mange. Mange is an animal disease in which the hair comes out in clumps.

Hypertrichosis is an abnormal condition of excessive hairiness. Hyper- = excessive + trich/o = hair + -osis = abnormal condition. A synonym is hirsutism.

A keratinous cyst is a benign cavity filled with epithelium that has become hardened (keratinized), sebum, and epithelial debris. A synonym for keratinous cyst is sebaceous cyst.

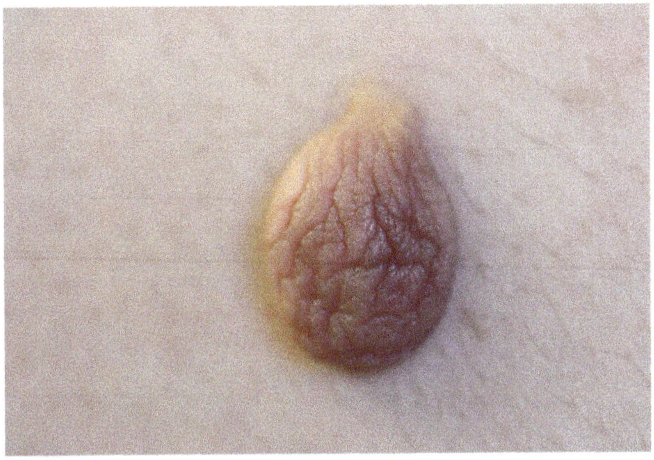

Verruca

Milia is a condition of tiny keratinous cysts that are on the surface of the skin. They are the result of clogged sebaceous ducts. Psoriasis is a common chronic skin disorder characterized by circumscribed salmon red patches covered by thick, dry, silvery scales.

Cornification means a process of becoming hard or horny (corne/o means hard, horny).

A callus is a thickening of the stratum corneum that occurs wherever there are areas of pressure or friction.

A corn (also called a clavus) is a mass of horny, condensed epithelial tissue that is over a bony prominence. It occurs as the result of pressure or friction.

A decubitus ulcer is an inflammation, sore, or erosion of the skin over a bony prominence. These occur most often in debilitated patients who are immobilized. These ulcers are graded by stages of severity, with the highest grade being a 4, describing one that is so deep that it has eroded tissue down to the bone. Note that other names for a decubitus ulcer are a pressure sore or pressure ulcer. You may have seen them referred to as bedsores.

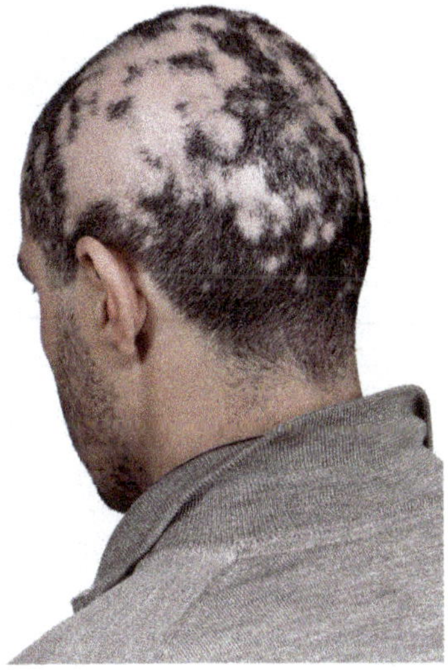

Alopecia

Ichthyosis is extremely dry skin. It is named by the combining form ichthy/o, meaning fish, because of the scaly appearance of the skin. A milder form of dry skin is xeroderma. Xer/o = dry.

Albinism is a condition of a lack of pigmentation in the skin. Albin/o is a combining form for white. Dyschromia (dys- = abnormal, chrom/o = color, and

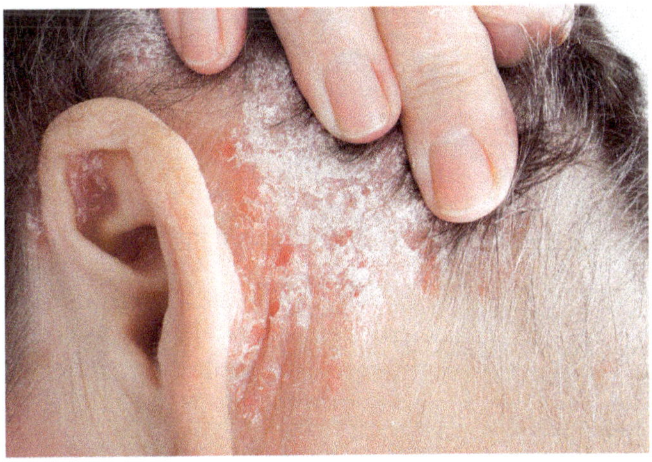

Psoriasis

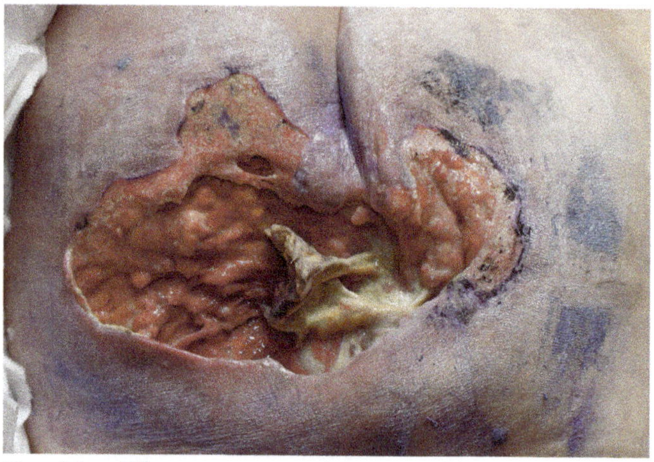

Decubitus Ulcer

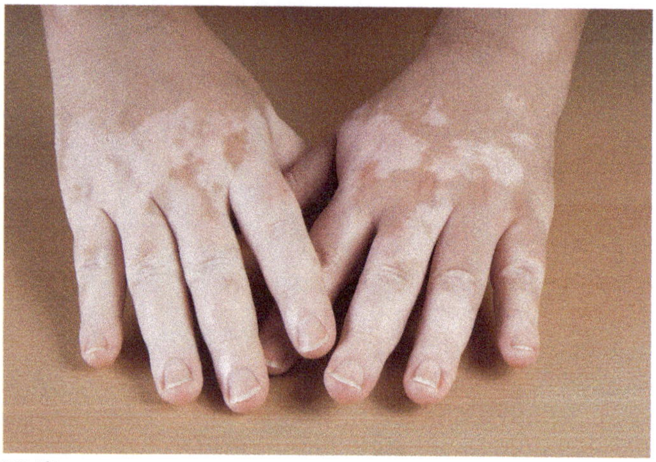

Vitiligo

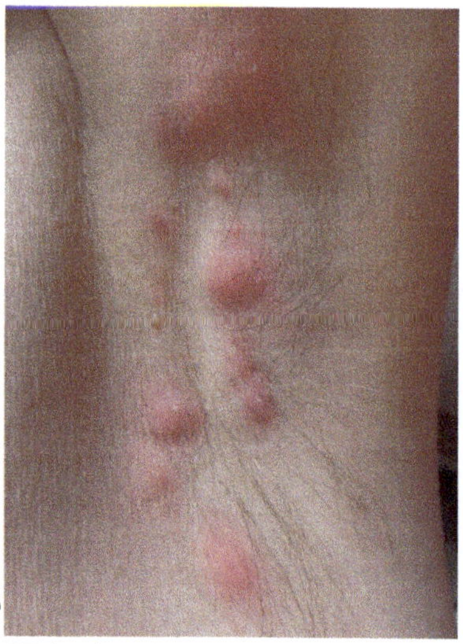

Hidradenitis

-ia = condition) is an abnormal condition of pigmentation of the skin. If an individual has less than normal pigmentation, it is referred to as hypochromia. If there is more than normal pigmentation, it is referred to as hyperchromia. Vitiligo is a condition of patches of skin that lack pigment as a result of an acquired disorder of unknown origin.

Anhidrosis is an abnormal condition of no sweating. An- = no, not, without + hidr/o = sweat + -osis = abnormal condition. Sweating is a mechanism to help control body temperature, if we are unable to sweat and control or cool down, our body would overheat with no way to cool off.

Hidradenitis is an inflammation of the sweat glands. Hidraden/o is a compound combining form built from hidr/o for sweat and aden/o, meaning gland. The suffix -itis means an inflammation.

Hyperhidrosis is an abnormal condition of excessive sweating. Hyper- means excessive and again hidr/o = sweat and -osis = abnormal condition.

Miliaria is a condition of occluded (blocked) sweat ducts.

There are also several terms that relate to disorders of the nails (both fingernails and toenails). Onychia is an inflammation of the nail. It is also called onychitis.

Onychocryptosis is an abnormal condition of an ingrown (crypt- means hidden) nail.

Onycholysis is a loosening or separation of the nail plate from the nail bed.

Onychomalacia is a softening of the nail. The suffix -malacia means a softening.

Onychomycosis is an abnormal condition of fungus of the nails. Myc/o means fungus.

Paronychia is an inflammation of the skin surrounding the nail. This can happen when an individual, for example, chews his or her cuticles and they become inflamed.

Burns can be caused by heat, radiation, chemicals, or electricity. We categorize burns based on severity. The severity is measured in degrees and thickness. Although many sources categorize burns in four degrees, we will only use three degrees of burns. If degrees are used, there are first-degree burns, which damage the epidermis only. First-degree burns are characterized by erythema (redness), tenderness, and hyperesthesia (hyper- = excessive + esthesi/o = feeling + -ia = condition), which is a heightened sensitivity to touch. Another name for a first-degree burn is a superficial burn.

Second-degree burns involve the epidermis and dermis, with erythema, vesicles, and the likelihood of scar formation. These are also called partial thickness burns. If the burn damages the top part of the dermis called the papillary layer, it is a superficial partial thickness burn. If the entire dermis is damaged (meaning that the reticular layer is included), it is referred to as a deep partial thickness burn.

Third-degree burns are those that damage the epidermis, dermis, and subcutaneous layer. Because the nerve endings in the dermis are destroyed, this type of burn does not cause pain. This is also called a full-thickness burn.

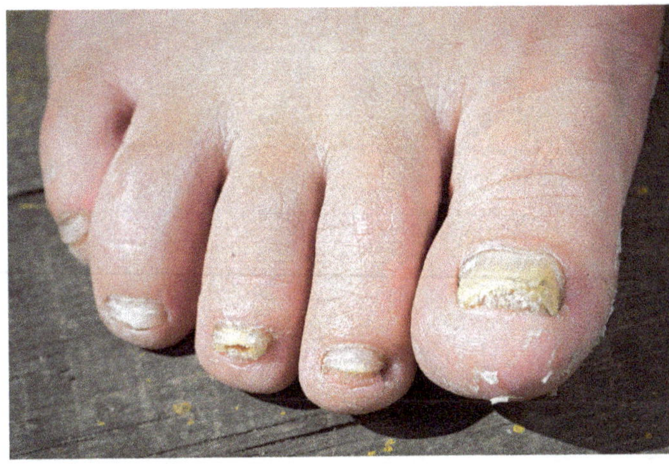

© Elena11/Shutterstock.com

Onychomycosis

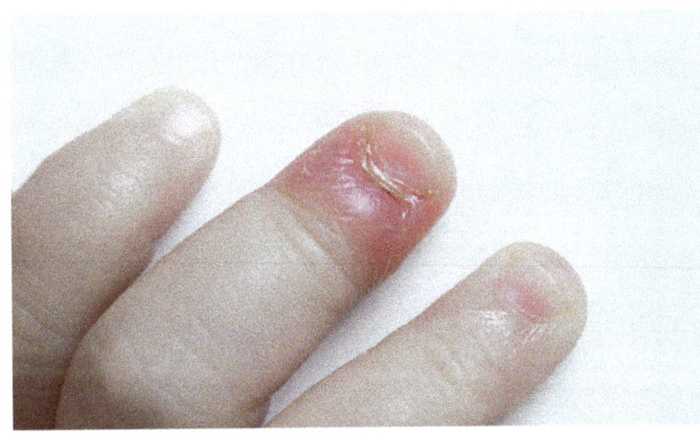

© zlikovec/Shutterstock.com

Paronychia

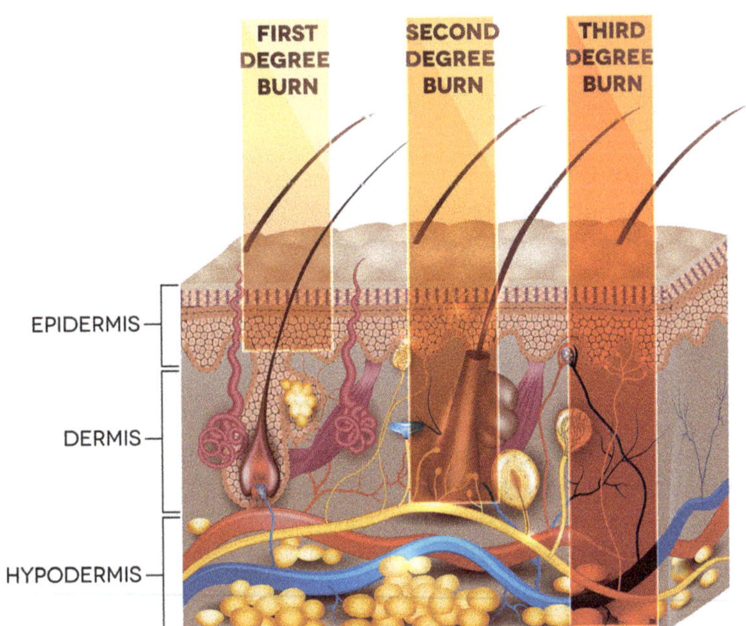

© Tefi/Shutterstock.com

Degrees of Burns

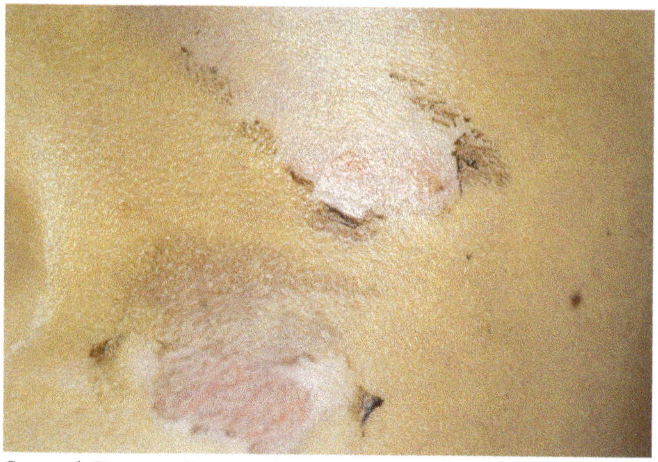

Second-Degree Burn

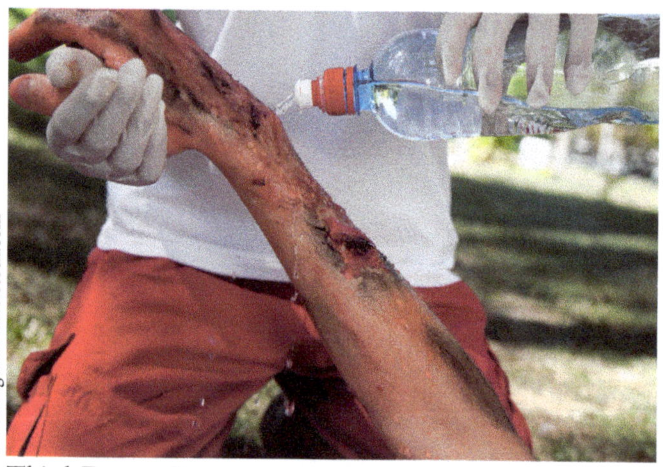

Third-Degree Burn

Eschar is the dried serum and blood that covers a burn.

The rule of nines is used to describe the percentage of the body that is affected by a burn by dividing the body into multiples of 9. As you can see, on the ventral surface of the body, 4.5% is allowed for the head and neck, 4.5% for each arm (9% total for the front of the arms), 18% for the front of the torso, 1% for the groin area, and 9% for each leg (18% total for the front of the legs). It gives us 50.5% for the front of the body. On the dorsal surface of the body, we again have 4.5% for the head and neck, 4.5% for the back of each arm (9%) total, 18% for the back of the torso, and 9% for the back of each leg (18% total for the legs). If the total back of the body is 49.5%, the total for the body is 100%.

Some patients need new skin after an injury, illness, or burn. In order for this to happen, the patient must have a skin graft. There are several different types of skin grafts.

A dermatome is an instrument to cut thin sheets of skin to be used for donor skin (dermat/o = skin + -tome = instrument to cut).

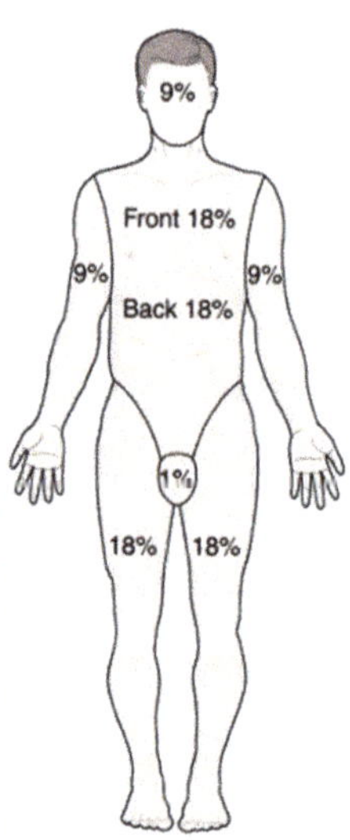

Rule of Nines

Sources of skin can be an autograft (NOT an autograph!), which is the skin that is taken from yourself (auto- = self). Skin for the face could be taken from an area that is not so visible, for example, the buttocks.

An allograft is skin that is taken from a donor of the same species (all/o = other), and a xenograft (xen/o = foreign) is a temporary skin graft that is taken from another species. A synonym for an allograft is a homograft, and a synonym for a xenograft is a heterograft (heter/o means different). A xenograft can be from a pig!

A flap is another term for a skin graft. These can be split-thickness, meaning that they are from the epidermis and part of the dermis. A full-thickness skin graft is from the entire epidermis and dermis.

Laser therapy is used to repair or destroy tissue, such as port wine stains, tattoos, or psoriatic lesions. Occlusive therapy is the use of a dressing that closes off (occlus/o = closing) an area of the skin to increase the effectiveness of the absorption and the effectiveness of a medication.

Psoralen plus ultraviolet A therapy is the use of ultraviolet light on psoriatic lesions.

Cauterization is the burning of tissues in order to destroy them. Cauter/i = burn.

Cryosurgery is the use of extreme cold (cry/o = extreme cold) to destroy lesions.

Curettage is the scraping of material from the wall of a cavity to obtain tissue for microscopic examination. The instrument used is a called a curette. Debridement is the first step in wound treatment; it is the process of removing dirt, foreign bodies, damaged tissue, and cellular debris from a wound or burn in order to prevent infection and promote healing.

An escharotomy is an incision to cut (and remove) eschar, the scab that forms over a burn; it is done to prevent edema that can cause a lack of blood flow (ischemia) to the underlying tissue. Incision and drainage (I&D) is the cutting open and the removal of the contents of a cyst, wound, or other lesion. Don't confuse this with ID, meaning intradermal (pertaining to within the skin). Mohs surgery is the repeated removal and microscopic examination of layers of a tumor until no cancerous cells are present.

Shaving/paring is the slicing of thin sheets of tissue to remove lesions.

If you need your eyelids "done," you would have a blepharoplasty. Blephar/o = eyelid + -plasty = surgical repair.

A chemical peel is the use of a mild acid to produce a superficial burn. This procedure is used to remove wrinkles and fine lines from the face.

Dermabrasion (-abrasion = scraping of) is a surgical procedure to resurface the skin. It is used to remove acne scars, moles (nevi), wrinkles, and tattoos.

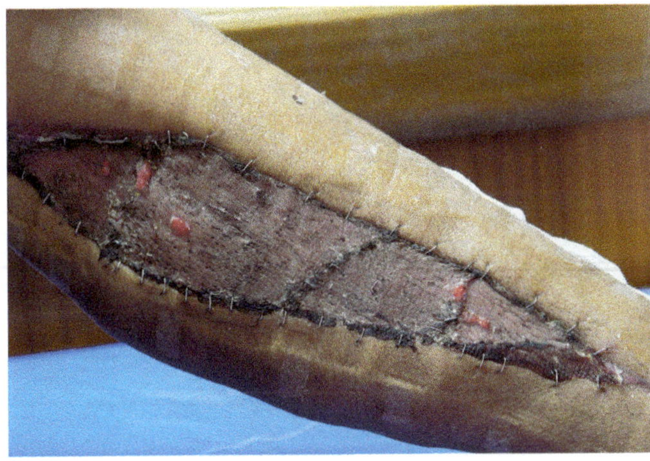

Skin Graft

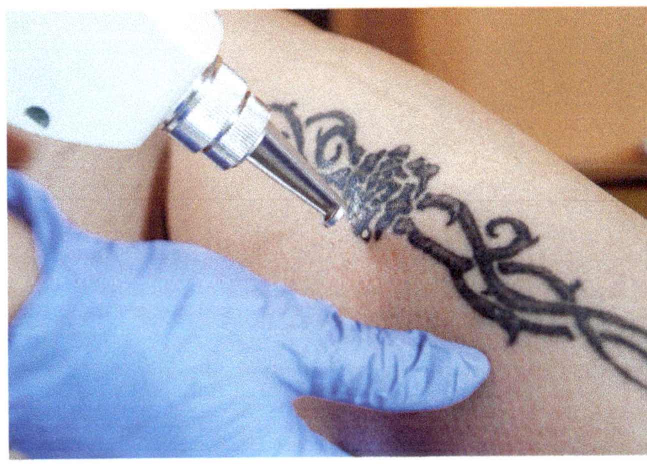

Laser Tattoo Removal

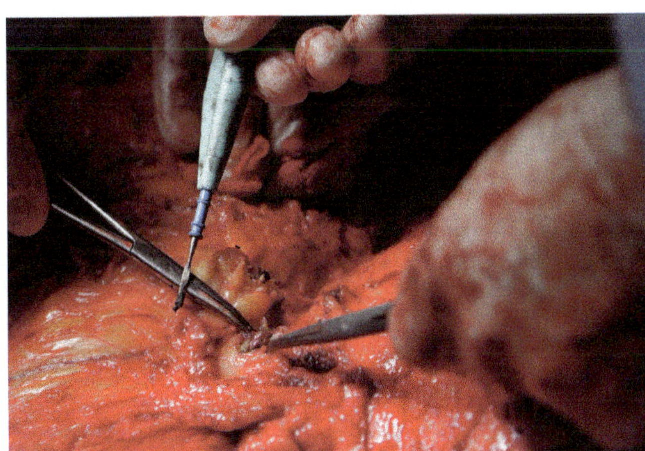

Cauterization

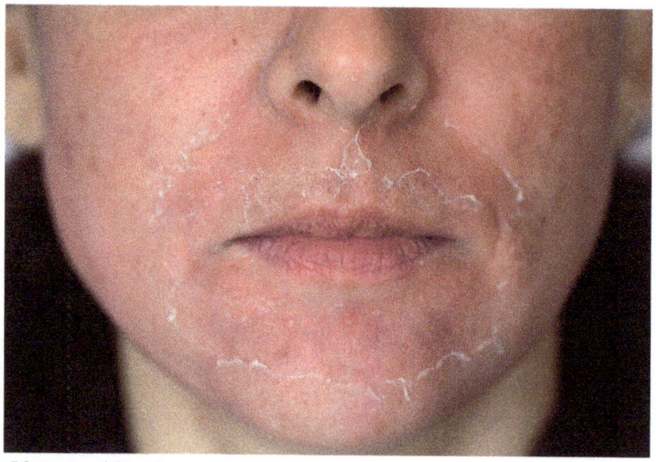

Chemical Peel

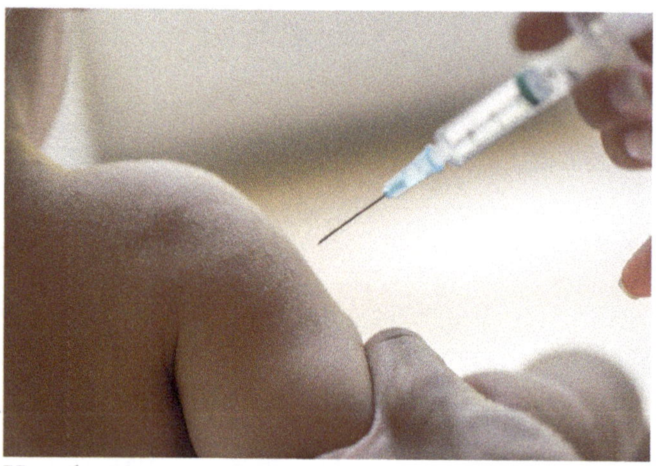

Hypodermic

Dermatoplasty, although literally the surgical repair of the skin, is the transplant of living skin to correct the effects of injury, operation, or disease.

A lipectomy is the removal (-ectomy) of fat (lip/o). Liposuction is a technique for removing excess adipose tissue with a suction pump device. A rhytidectomy (rhytid/o = wrinkle) is a surgical procedure to remove wrinkles. This is commonly known as a facelift.

For medications to be administered either on, in, under, or through the skin, we use different methods. The skin is the primary protective barrier. We use different methods to administer medications in varying doses and routes.

Hypodermic means pertaining to under (hypo-) the skin. Subcutaneous also means pertaining to under (sub-) the skin. Intradermal means pertaining to within (intra-) the skin.

Topical is a type of drug that is applied directly onto the skin. It could be a cream, gel, lotion, or ointment. A transdermal therapeutic system delivers medication through (trans-) the skin using a patch that allows for a specified time release of a medication.

There are many medications that we give in the different ways listed.

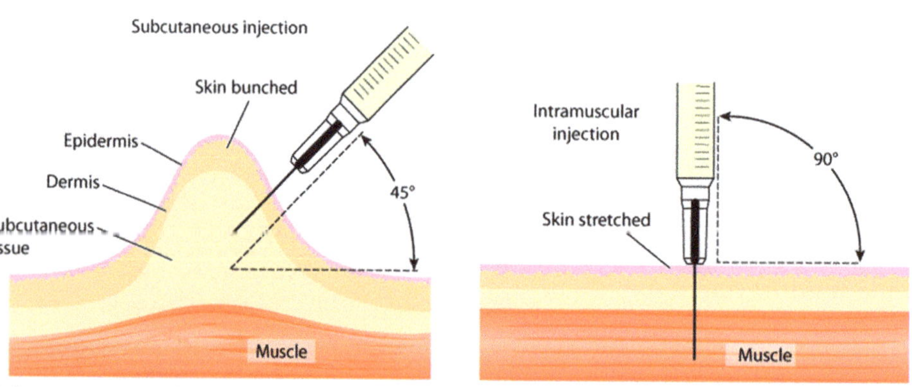

Subcutaneous and Intramuscular

These medications treat the skin and body in different ways. Some examples of these medication types are anesthetic, antibacterial, antifungal, antihistamine, and antiinflammatory.

Anesthetic agents are drugs to reduce pain and discomfort; they can be given topically on an affected area. Examples include lidocaine (Solarcaine) and benzocaine (Orajel).

Antibacterials are drugs that prevent and treat bacterial growth. Examples are bacitracin, Silvadene, erythromycin, and tetracycline.

Antifungals are drugs that attack fungi. Examples are Lotromin, Nystat, and Spectazole.

Antihistamines are drugs that decrease itching by reducing an allergic response. Examples are Benadryl, Chlor-Trimetron, Zyrtec, and Claritin.

Antiinflammatories are used to reduce inflammation and pain. Examples are Cortizone, Lidex, and Kenalog.

More pharmacology:

Antipsoriatics are agents that specifically treat psoriasis, such as Drithocreme and Dovonex.

Antiseptics are topical agents used to prevent infection by destroying microbials. Iodine and Peridex are examples.

Antivirals are drugs that are designed to decrease the effect of viruses, such as Valtrex and Zovirax.

Emollients are topical substances that soften the skin. Lubriderm is a well-known example.

Immunomodulators or immunosuppressants are agents that suppress the body's immune system. Elidel and Protopic are examples of drugs that are used to treat atopic dermatitis and eczema.

Keratolytics are topical substances used to break down hardened skin and shed the top layer of dead skin. They are used to treat warts, calluses, corns, acne, and psoriasis. Examples are salicylic acid, Benzac, and Condylox.

The skin is the largest organ in the body and a complex system of tissue. We must be diligent to understand the basis of Chapters 1 and 2 in order to begin to dissect the words in the integumentary system.

CHAPTER 4

Skeletal

The bones are the primary organs of the skeletal system. There are 206 bones in the body that, along with cartilage, tendons, and ligaments, make up the framework of the body. We will divide the skeleton into two parts; axial and appendicular. The axial skeleton is made up of the skull, spine, ribs, and sternum. The axial skeleton has 80 bones. The appendicular skeleton is made up of the shoulder, arms, hands, pelvic, legs, and feet. The appendicular skeleton has 126 bones. Interestingly enough bones are made up of 50% water and 50% solid matter.

The functions of the skeletal system are:

- Acting as a framework for the organ systems,
- Protecting many of the body's organs,
- Providing the organism with the ability to move,
- Storing minerals, and
- Hematopoiesis.

The chest cavity provides a framework as well as protects the heart, lungs, esophagus, and trachea. The bones act as a type of "bank" for the minerals. The body stores and makes the withdrawals of minerals such as calcium and phosphorus in the bones. The formation of blood is hematopoiesis, a function provided by the bone marrow. Hemat/o = blood and -poiesis = formation.

The musculoskeletal system (MS) is composed of bones, muscles, and joints. Joints are sometimes referred to as articulations. Be careful! The abbreviation MS also stands for mitral stenosis and multiple sclerosis. The bones are connected by fibrous bands of tissue called ligaments. Muscles are connected to bones by tendons. The tough outer covering of the muscles is the fascia. The articular cartilage is the covering of the ends of many bones and also serves as a protective function.

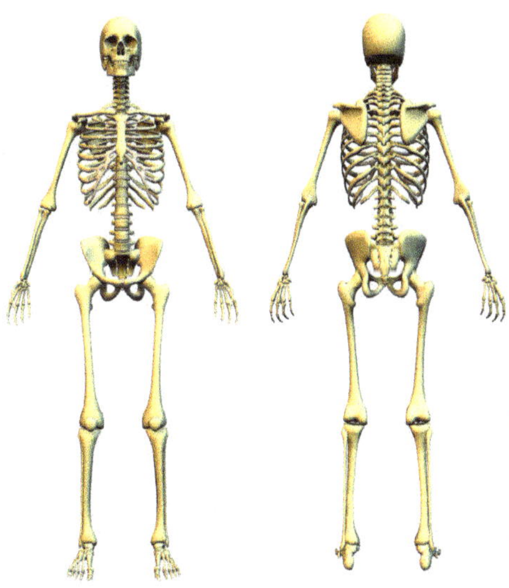

Skeleton

Bones (oste/o, oss/i, osse/o)
Muscles (muscul/o, my/o, myos/o)
Joints/articulations (arthr/o, articul/o)

Ligaments (ligament/o, syndesm/o)
Tendons (tendin/o, tend/o, ten/o)
Fascia (fasci/o)
Cartilage (cartilag/o, chondr/o)

There are also different types and different shapes of bones.

- Long bones
- Short bones
- Flat bones
- Irregular bones
- Sesamoid bones

Examples of long bones are the femur (thighbone) and the humerus (upper arm bone). Some short bones are the carpals (wrist bones) and tarsals (ankle bones), flat bones are the sternum (breastbone)

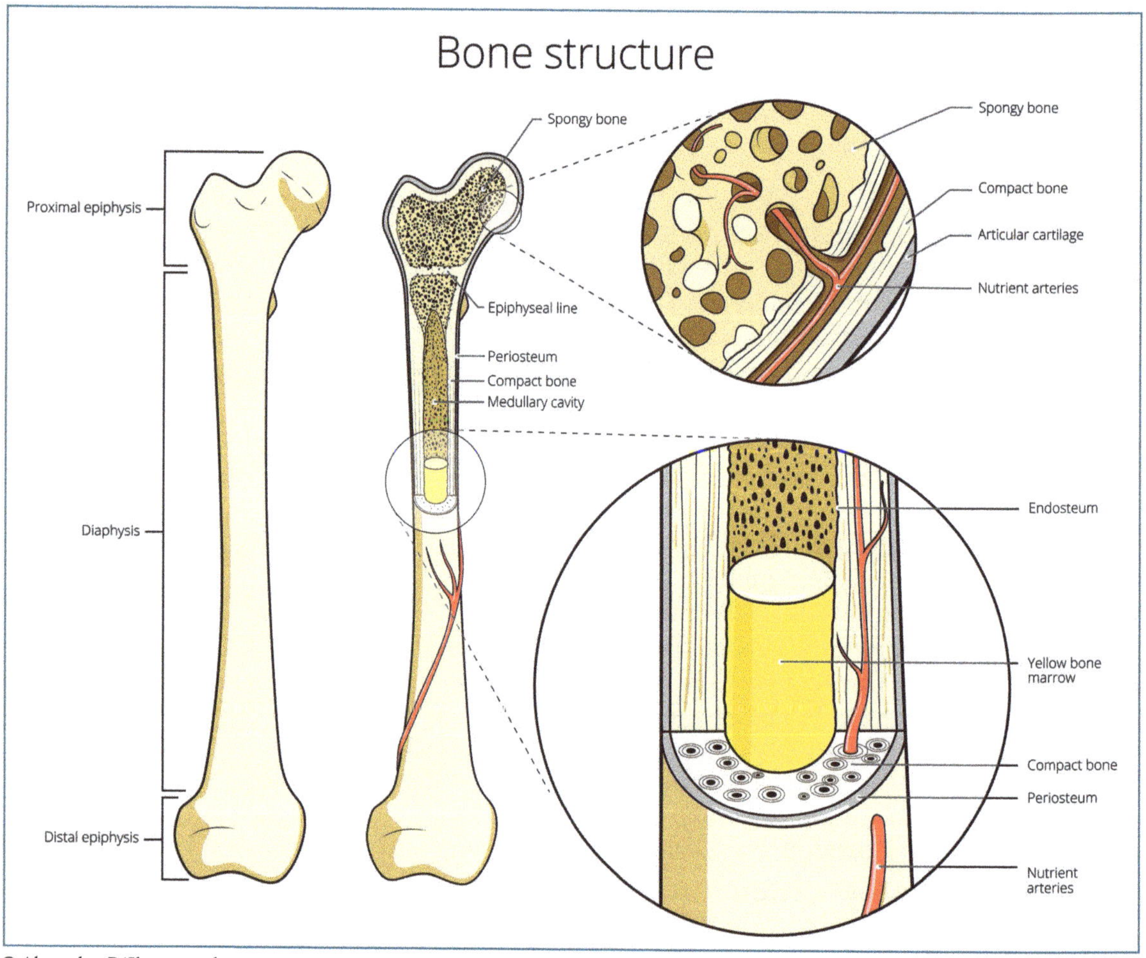

and the scapula (shoulder blade), and irregular bones are the vertebrae (back bones). The final group of bones are the sesamoid bones and one of the examples for these bones is the patella (knee cap).

Bones are built from mature bone cells called osteocytes (oste/o = bone + -cyte = cell) and the substance between them called the matrix. Immature bone cells called osteoblasts (oste/o = bone + -blast = embyonic) are cells that build bone, while osteoclasts (oste/o = bone + -clast = breaking down) break down bone cells to use them as needed.

The osteocytes and the matrix make up the hard outer layer called compact bone. Underneath the compact bone is the cancellous bone (also called spongy bone, which is also composed of osteocytes and matrix, but not as dense as the compact bone). Inside of the spongy bone are the medullary cavity and the red bone marrow, which produces the blood cells for the body.

Each long bone is composed of a shaft, termed the diaphysis (dia- = through, complete + -physis = growth) and the ends of the bone called the epiphyses (s. epiphysis). The prefix epi-, meaning above, indicates that this structure is above the ends of the bone. The epiphyseal plate is the area where the bone growth normally occurs. Around age 16, the epiphyseal plates close and bone growth stops. The metaphysis (meta- means change) is the area of both the epiphysis and the epiphyseal plate. The periosteum (peri- = surrounding, oste/o = bone + -um = structure) is the structure surrounding bone, and the endosteum (endo- = within) is the structure within bone.

Bone depressions are grooves, openings, or hollow spaces that provide protection. These also allow an entrance and exit point for blood vessels and/or nerves and hold organs or glands. A foramen is an opening in a bone. A fossa is a hollow or a depression in bone. A sinus (also called an antrum) is a cavity within bone.

Foramen (pl. foramina) (foramin/o)
Fossa (pl. fossae) (foss/o)
Sinus (pl. sinuses) (sinus/o, sin/o)

Bone processes are the opposite of bone depressions. They are projections that protrude from bone, usually serving as points of attachment for ligaments and tendons. There are several terms that are associated with these projections:

A condyle is a rounded projection at the end of bone.

A crest is a narrow elongated elevation.

An epicondyle is a projection on the surface of bone above a condyle.

A bone head is a rounded, usually proximal portion of some long bones.

A spine is a thornlike projection.

A trochanter is one of two bony projections on the proximal ends of the femurs that serve as points of attachment for muscles.

A tubercle is a nodule or small raised area.

A tuberosity is an elevation or protuberance, which is larger than a tubercle.

Condyle (condyl/o)
Crest
Epicondyle (epicondyl/o)

Head
Spine (spin/o)
Trochanter (trochanter/o)
Tubercle (tubercul/o)
Tuberosity

The skull: cranial bone is made up of the cranium and the facial bones. The cranium is made up of the frontal bone, which forms the anterior part of the skull and the forehead. The parietal bones, which form the sides of the skull. The occipital bone, which forms the back of the skull. This bone contains the foramen magnum, which allows the brain communication with the spinal cord. The temporal bones, which form the lower two sides of the cranium. The mastoid process is the posterior part of the temporal bone that is behind the ear. The ethmoid bone forms the roof and the walls of the nasal cavity. The sphenoid bone is anterior to the temporal bones and is the basilar part of the occipital bone. The zygomatic bones are the cheekbones. The lacrimal bones are paired bones at the corner of each eye that cradle the tear ducts. The maxilla is the upper jaw bone. The mandible is the lower jaw bone.

Zygoma (zygom/o, zygomat/o)
Lacrimal bones (lacrim/o)
Maxilla (maxill/o)
Mandible (mandibul/o)

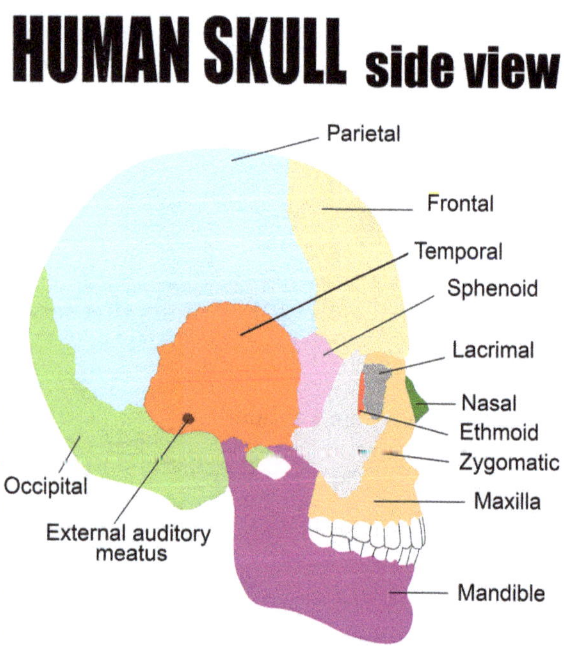

Bones of the Skull

There are 12 pairs of ribs. These bones are flat and attached to the thoracic vertebrae in the back and to the constochondral tissue in the front. There are seven pairs of true ribs that are attached directly to the breastbone (the sternum). There are five pairs of false ribs that are attached to the sternum by cartilage. There are two floating ribs that are not attached in the front of the body at all. The medical term for the breastbone is the sternum (stern/o).

The thin plates that protrude in a posterior fashion from the vertebra are spinous processes. The ones that extend in a lateral direction are transverse processes. The arches between the transverse processes and the spinous processes are termed the laminae (s. lamina). The main part of the back bone is called the vertebral body. There are seven cervical vertebrae (cervic/o = neck), twelve thoracic vertebrae (thorac/o = chest), five lumbar vertebrae

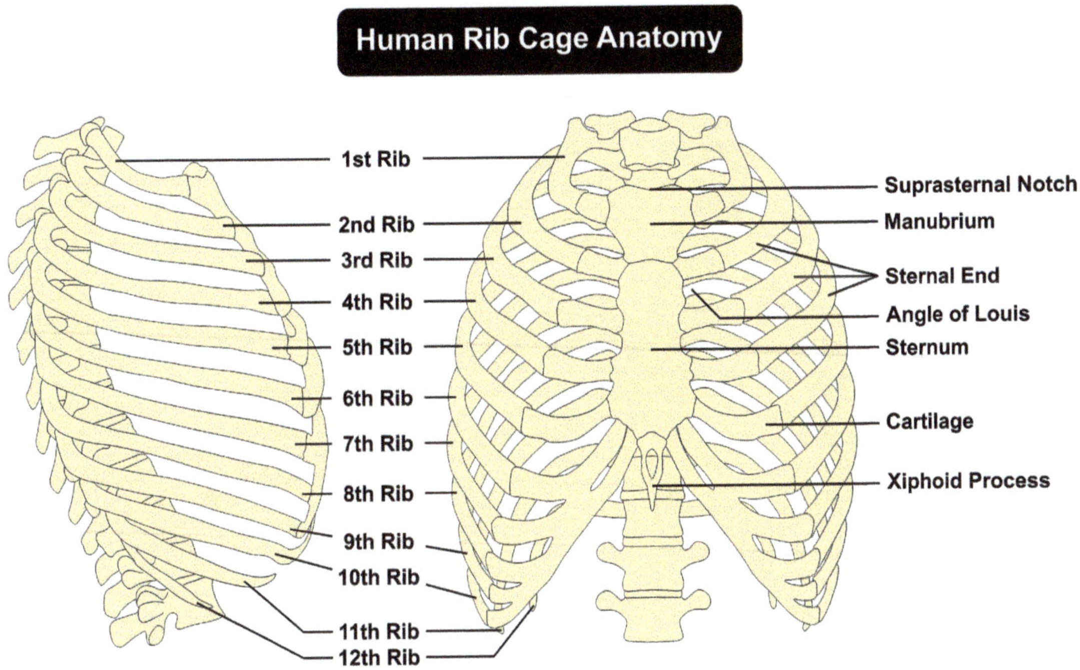

© udaix/Shutterstock.com

(lumb/o = lumbar), five fused sacral vertebrae (sacr/o = sacrum), and finally the tail bone, which is called the coccyx (or coccygeal vertebrae).

Cervical C1–C7 (cervic/o)
Thoracic T1–T12 (thorac/o)
Lumbar L1–L5 (lumb/o)
Sacral S1–S5 (sacr/o)
Coccygeal (coccyg/o)

The upper portion of the appendicular skeleton (basically from the shoulder to the tips of the fingers) consists of the following bones:

The scapulae are the shoulder blades, which are flat bones on the dorsal aspect of the body. The acromion process is the lateral protrusion of the scapula that forms the highest point of the shoulder. The clavicles are the collarbones. These are long, curved horizontal bones that attach to the upper sternum at one end and to the acromion process of the scapula at the other. These bones help stabilize the shoulder in the front of the body. The humerus is the upper arm bone. The radius is the lower lateral arm bone (remember to position the body in anatomical position to determine which bone is medial and which is lateral). The ulna is the lower medial arm bone. The olecranon is a proximal projection of the ulna that forms the tip of the elbow. This "funny bone" is actually a process, not a separate bone. The carpal bones are those of the wrist. The metacarpal bones are the hand bones. The phalanges are the bones of the fingers and toes. Ask the class how many bones are

The structure of the segments of the spine

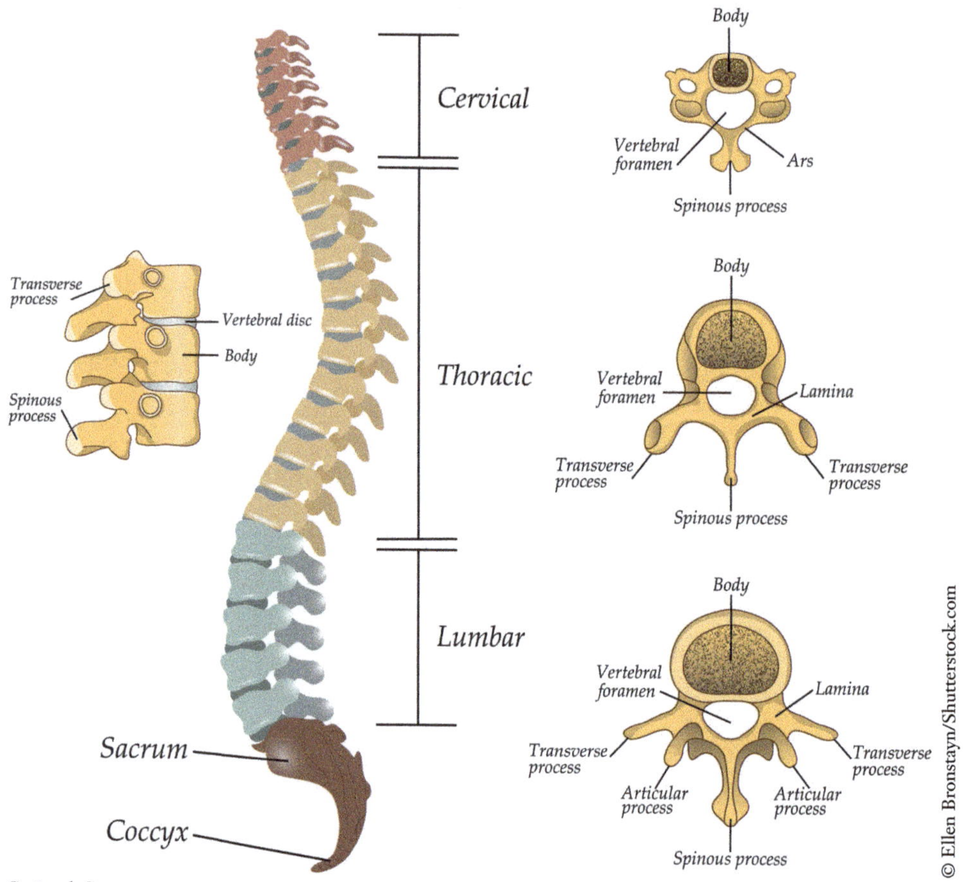

Spinal Segments

in the thumb or great toe (two in each) or in each of the fingers or toes (three each). The term for a whole finger or toe is a digitus.

Scapula (scapul/o)
Clavicle (clavicul/o, cleid/o)
Humerus (humer/o)
Radius and ulna (radi/o, uln/o)
Carpus (carp/o)
Metacarpus (metacarp/o)
Phalanges (phalang/o)

The lower portion of the appendicular skeleton (basically from the pelvis to the tips of the toes) consists of the following bones:

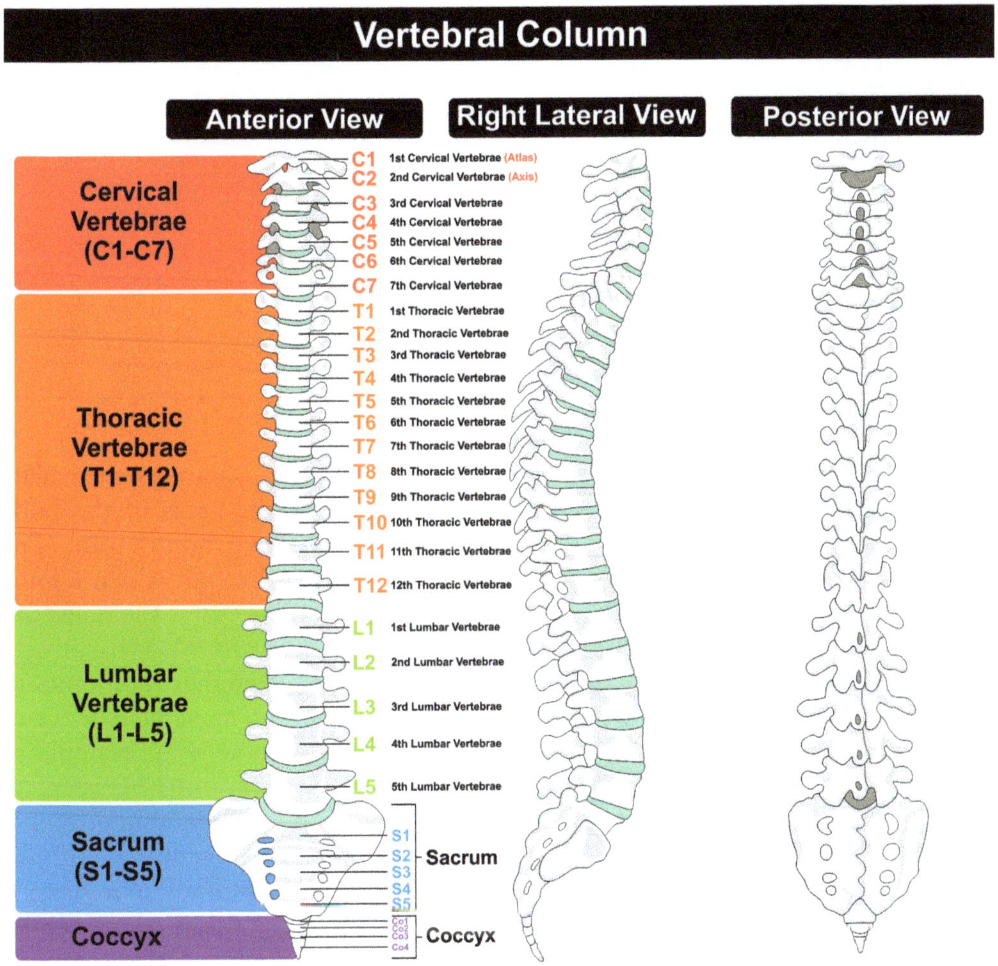

The bones in the pelvis are the ilium, the superior and widest bone; the ischium, the lower portion of the pelvis; and the pubis, the lower anterior bone of the pelvis. Note that the pelvis is instrumental in determining the sex of a skeleton (an angle of the bones at the pubis greater than 90 degrees usually indicates a female). In the leg, the thigh bone is the femur. The kneecap is the patella, the shin bone is the tibia, and the lower lateral leg bone is the fibula. The distal processes of the tibia and fibula are the medial and lateral malleoli (s. malleolus). The bones of the ankle are the tarsals, while the bones of the foot are the metatarsals. The heelbone is the calcaneus. As with the fingers, the bones of the toes are termed phalanges (s. phalanx).

Pelvis

- (pelv/i, pelv/o)
- Ilium (ili/o)
- Ischium (ischi/o)
- Pubis (pub/o)

Leg

- Femur (femor/o)
- Patella (patell/o, patell/a)
- Tibia (tibi/o)
- Fibula (fibul/o, perone/o)
- Tarsus (tars/o)
- Metatarsus (metatars/o)
- Phalanges (phalang/o)

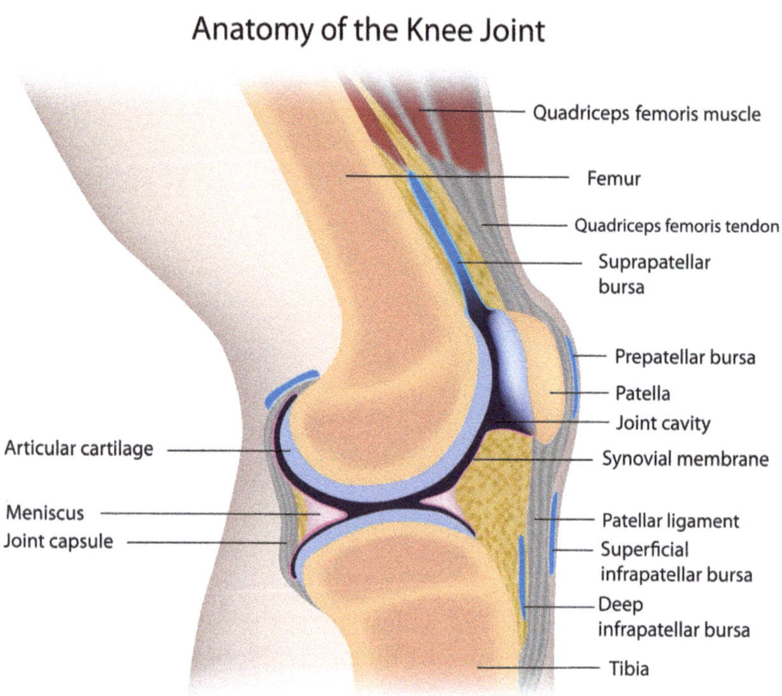

Joints, or articulations, are the areas of the body where two bones join. The range through which a joint can be moved is the range of motion, or ROM. Synarthroses (syn- = together) are joints that have no movement because they are joined. An example would be the joints between the bones of the cranium. Amphiarthroses (amphi- = both) are joints that have limited motion, such as the vertebrae or the pubic bones. Diarthroses, also called synovial joints, are joints that have free movement. The prefix di- means through, indicating that the joint is able to move through its range of motion freely. Examples are the knees, shoulders, and ankles. Synovial joints have joint capsules that enclose the ends of the bones and a synovial membrane that lines the joint capsules and secretes fluid to lubricate the joint. Bursae are sacs of fluid that are located between the bones of the joint and provide a cushioning function. Along with the cushioning that bursae provide, articular cartilage covers and protects the ends of the bone, and the meniscus is a crescent-shaped cartilage in the knee joint that additionally cushions the joint.

Attached to the skeletal structure are muscles. These muscles have the ability to contract and relax. Skeletal muscle is voluntary in nature and striated in appearance. Smooth muscle is what the organs are composed of and is involuntary in nature. Heart muscle has unique properties that keep the heart beating without rest. Tendons are the bands of tissue that connect muscles to bones. These bands have an origin (where the bone at the end of the attachment does not move and is nearest to the trunk) and an insertion (the end of bone that does move and is farthest from the trunk).

Antagonistic muscles are those that work against each other in pairs in order to carry out a movement. For example, one set of muscles must contract while the other set relaxes in order to flex or extend a limb.

Synergistic muscles are those that work together to refine a movement.

The sternocleidomastoid muscle is a term that is built out of three word parts. Sterno meaning sternum, where the muscle attaches to the sternum. Cleido meaning clavicle, where it also attaches to the clavicle. Finally, we have mastoid, where the muscle attaches to the mastoid process, which is the lower part of the mastoid bone.

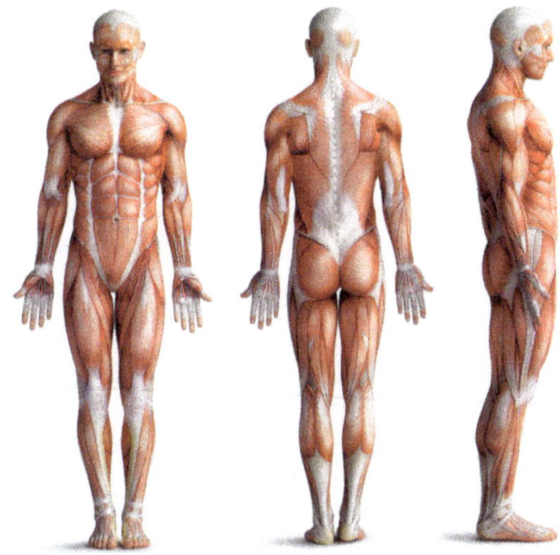

Muscles

© adike/Shutterstock.com

All muscle have actions. Some of those actions involve being able to contract and relax. We give specific names to these actions. When working in pairs, one set relaxes while the other contracts in order to pull limbs into a variety of positions. The action of extension is the process of stretching out, of increasing the angle of a joint. Flexion is the process of decreasing the angle of a joint. Adduction means toward the midline and abduction means away from the midline. An easy way to remember these is adduction is adding back toward the body. Abduction is being taken away from the body. Supination is the process of turning the palm or medial side of the foot upward. Pronation is the process of turning the palm or medial side of the foot downward. Dorsiflexion is the process of bending back. Plantar flexion is the action of lowering the foot, pointing the toes away from the shin. Eversion is the process of turning a body part outward, while inversion is the process of turning the body part inward. Rotation is the process of a bone turning on its axis (like a wheel), while circumduction is a circular movement of the distal end of a limb around its point of attachment. Mostly everyone has some ability to rotate their head but circumduction of the head is impossible. Protraction (pro = forward + tract/o = pulling + -ion = process of) is the forward movement of a muscle, while retraction (re- = backward) is the backward movement of a muscle.

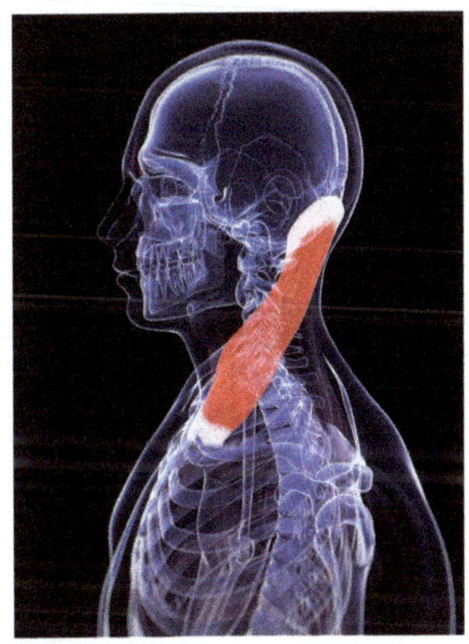

Sternocleidomastoid Muscle

© Sebastian Kaulitzki/Shutterstock.com

Polydactyly (poly- = many, much + dactyl/o = fingers/toes + -y = process of) is a condition of more than five fingers or toes on each hand or foot. Syndactyly (syn- = joined, together) is a condition of the joining of the fingers

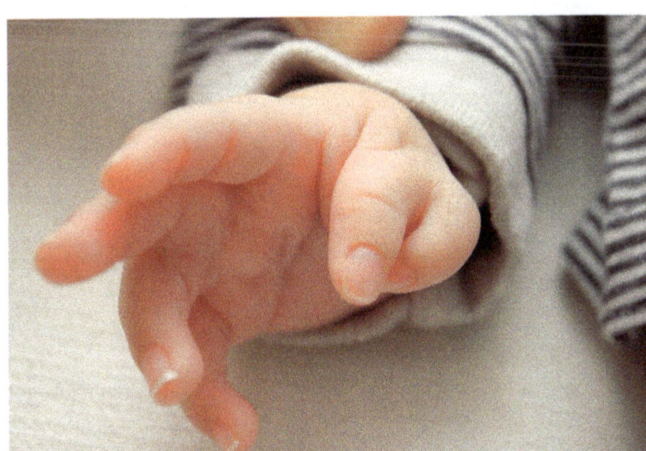

Polydactyly

© v.gi/Shutterstock.com

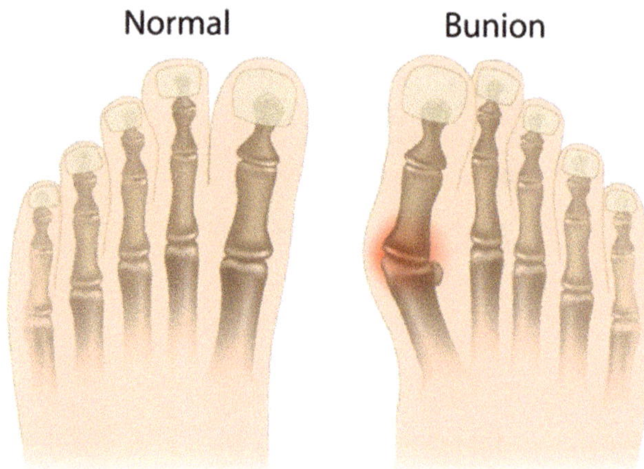

Bunion

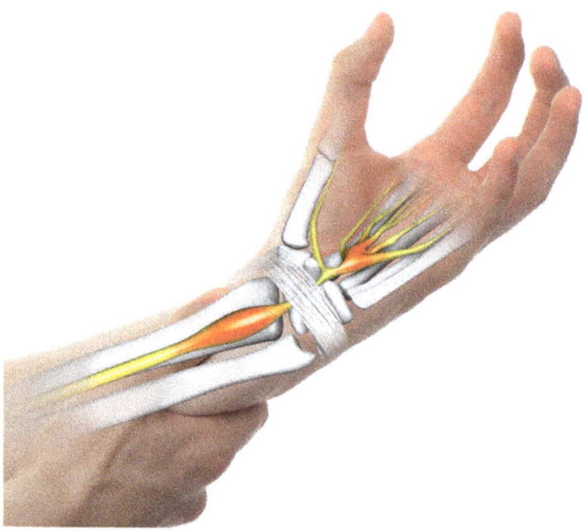

Carpal Tunnel

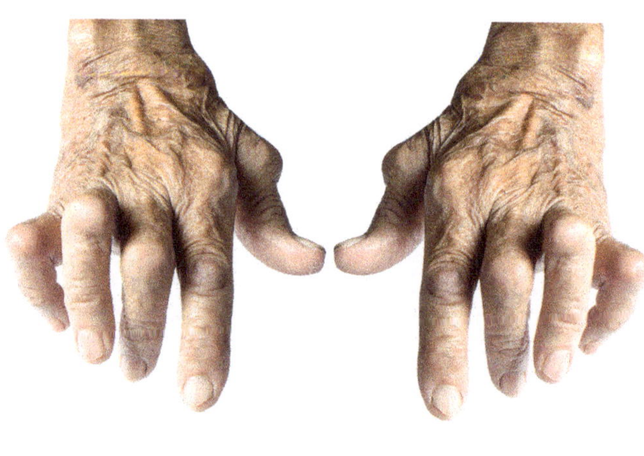

Rheumatoid Arthritis

or toes, giving them a webbed appearance. Spina bifida occulta (bi- = two + -fida = split + occulta = hidden) is a congenital malformation of the bony spinal canal without involvement of the spinal cord.

Osteodynia (-dynia = pain) is a term for bone pain. Osteitis deformans is a term for misshapen bone as a result of inflammation. Osteomalacia (-malacia = softening) is a softening of the bone. This is usually caused by a loss of minerals in the bony matrix as a result of a vitamin D deficiency. If the disorder occurs in childhood, it is called rickets. Osteomyelitis is inflammation of the bone and bone marrow. Osteoporosis is the loss of bone mass (por/o = passages), which results in the bones being fragile and at risk for fractures. A lesser condition is osteopenia (-penia = deficiency), where there is a loss of bone mass, but it is not as severe as osteoporosis.

A bunion is a common, painful enlargement and inflammation of the first metatarsophalangeal joint (the base of the great toe). Carpal tunnel syndrome (CTS) is a compression injury that manifests itself as fluctuating pain, numbness, and paresthesias (abnormal sensations like prickling) of the hand caused by the compression of the median nerve at the wrist. Temporomandibular joint disorder (TMJ) is a dysfunctional joint between the lower jaw bone and the temporal bone of the skull. It may be accompanied by gnathalgia, which is pain of the jaw (gnath/o = jaw).

Osteoarthritis is a joint disease that is characterized by degenerative articular cartilage and a wearing down of the edges of the bone at the joint. A synonym for osteoarthritis is degenerative joint disease. Rheumatoid arthritis is an autoimmune inflammatory joint disease, which usually occurs in a much younger population (20–45) than osteoarthritis.

Arthrosis is any abnormal condition of a joint (-osis = abnormal condition). Specific types of arthroses are

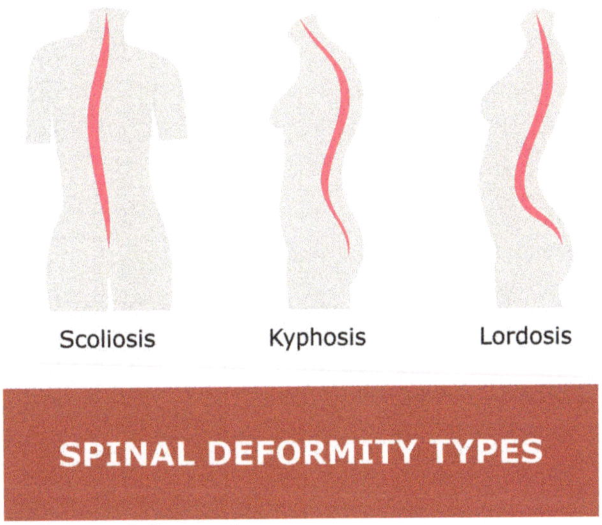

© Pawel Graczyk/Shutterstock.com

hemarthrosis (hem/o = blood), an abnormal condition of blood in a joint; hydrarthrosis (hydr/o = water, fluid), an abnormal condition of fluid in a joint; and pyarthrosis (py/o = pus), an abnormal condition of pus in a joint. A Baker cyst is a small sac (a cyst) filled with synovial fluid in the popliteal area of the leg (back of the knee). It is often associated with rheumatoid arthritis. Bursitis is an inflammation of a bursa. It may be caused by overuse of a joint. Crepitus is a crackling sound that may be heard in the joints. Osteophytosis (phyt/o = growth) is an abnormal condition of bony growths in a joint. Heberden nodes are osteophytes of the interphalangeal joints in rheumatoid arthritis. Scleroderma (scler/o—hard) is a connective tissue disorder that causes hardening and thickening of the skin. Systemic lupus erythematosus (erythemato/o = red) is a chronic systemic disorder characterized by a distinctive butterfly rash on the nose and cheeks. Tendinitis is an inflammation of a tendon.

Dorsalgia is a term that is used to describe upper back pain (dors/o = back + -algia = pain). Lumbago is used to describe lower back pain (lumb/o = lumbar + -ago = disease). Sometimes, the normal slight curvatures of the spine are exaggerated and cause pain or dysfunction for a patient. Hence, each of these terms for malcurvatures ends with the suffix -osis for an abnormal condition. Scoliosis (scoli/o = curvature) is a lateral S curve of the spine. This condition can literally cause an individual to lose inches in height. Lordosis (lord/o = swayback) is an exaggerated anterior curve of the lumbar vertebrae. Kyphosis (kyph/o = roundback) is an extreme posterior curvature of the thoracic area of the spine.

A contracture is chronic fixation of a joint in flexion. This is caused by atrophy and shortening of the muscle fibers after a long period of disuse. Fibromyalgia (fibr/o = fiber + my/o = muscle + -algia = pain) is a disorder that is characterized by musculoskeletal pain, fatigue, muscle stiffness and spasms, and sleep disturbances. Myasthenia gravis (my/o = muscle + a- = without, no + -sthenia = condition of strength, gravis means severe) is a usually serious condition that is characterized by fatigue and progressive muscle weakness, especially of the face and throat. Plantar fasciitis is an inflammation of the fascia (covering of the muscles) on the bottom of the foot. Polymyositis (poly- = many + my/o = muscle + -itis = inflammation) is a chronic, idiopathic inflammation of several voluntary muscles. Postlaminectomy syndrome (post- = after + lamin/o = lamina + -ectomy = removal) is a group of symptoms that occur together after the removal of a lamina to correct a spinal disorder. Rhabdomyolysis (rhabdomy/o = striated muscle + -lysis = breakdown, destruction) is the breakdown of striated/skeletal muscle.

Fractures, sprains, strains, dislocations, and subluxations make trauma pathology. Closed fractures (also called simple fractures) are those in which the bone is broken, but the skin remains intact. Open fracture (also called compound fractures) are those in which the bone is broken and one or both ends pierce the skin. A pathologic fracture is one that results from an underlying disease, such as osteoporosis or cancer. A synonym is a spontaneous fracture. Comminuted fractures are those in which the bone is crushed and/or shattered into multiple pieces. A compression fracture is one in which the

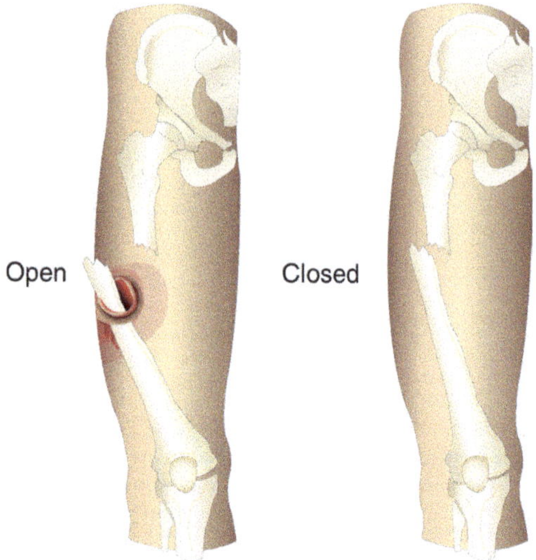

Open vs Closed Fracture

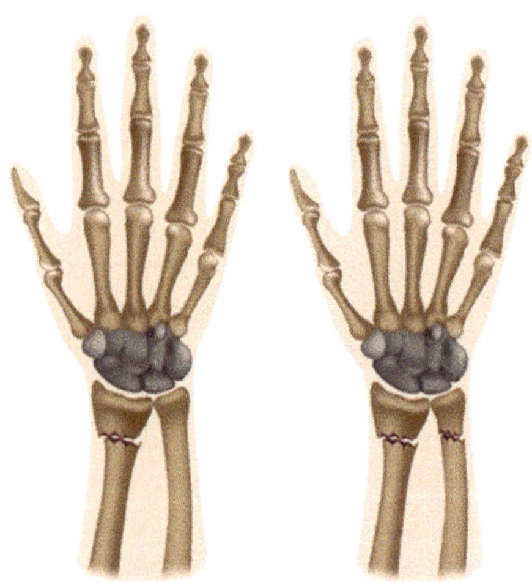

bone collapses on itself. A complicated fracture is one in which the bone is broken and one or both ends then pierce an internal organ. An example would be a broken rib that then pierces a lung or the heart. A Colles' fracture occurs at the distal end of the radius at the epiphysis. It usually occurs as a result of bracing oneself for a fall.

An impacted fracture is one in which the ends of the broken bones are driven into each other. A hairline fracture is a minor fracture appearing as a thin line on an x-ray. This type of fracture may or may not extend through the bone. A greenstick fracture is one in which the bone is partially bent and partially broken. It is relatively common in children because their bones are still somewhat soft. A Salter Harris fracture occurs at the epiphyseal plate in children.

A sprain is a traumatic injury to a joint that involves the ligaments. The severity of a sprain is measured in grades. A strain is a lesser injury that involves the overuse or over stretching of a muscle or tendon. A dislocation occurs when a bone is completely out of its place in a joint. If it is a partial dislocation, it is termed a subluxation. Compartment syndrome is a potentially serious medical condition that is the result of swelling within the fascia. The increased pressure of the swelling limits the blood supply, which can lead to nerve and muscle damage.

Therapeutic interventions can be defined as something that heals or assists in healing and helping someone with a disease or ailment. There are many different interventions for the skeletal system.

An amputation is the removal of a limb when there are no feasible options to save it. An artificial body part that is constructed to replace missing limbs, eyes, and other body parts is called a prosthesis (pl. prostheses). The removal of a bunion is a bunionectomy (-ectomy = removal). Osteoclasis is the refracture of a bone (oste/o = bone + -clasis = intentional breaking). This may be necessary if a malunion has occurred. Osteoplasty is surgical repair of a bone (-plasty = surgical repair). Traction is the process of pulling a body part into correct alignment, as in the correction of a dislocation. Kyphoplasty is a minimally invasive procedure designed to address the pain of fractured vertebrae resulting from osteoporosis or cancer. Kyph/o = round back (as in kyphosis), which may be caused by a loss of bone mass. A balloon is used to inflate the area of the fracture, and a cementlike substance is injected. A laminectomy is the removal of the bony arches of one or more vertebrae to relieve compression of the spinal cord. Spondylosyndesis (spondyl/o = vertebra + syn-= together + -desis = binding) is a fixation of an unstable segment of the spine using spinal traction, a body cast, or stabilization with a bone graft or synthetic device. Synonyms are spinal fusion and spondylodesis.

TYPES OF BONE FRACTURES

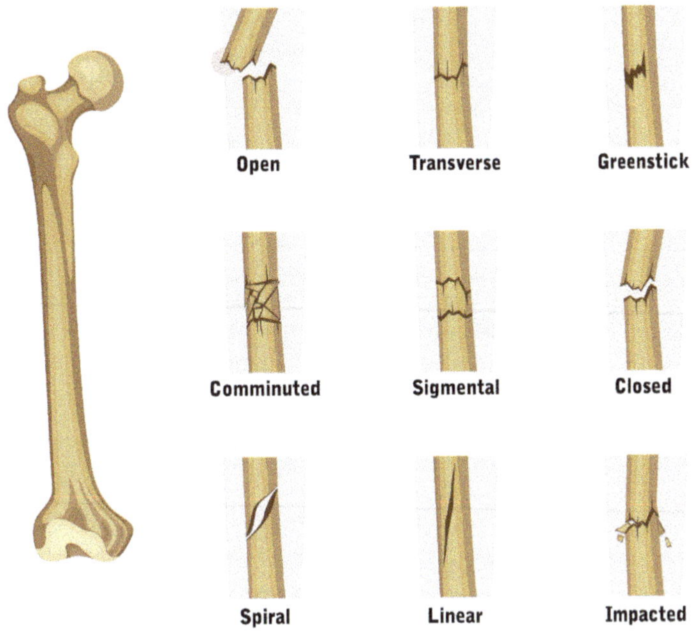

© logika600/Shutterstock.com

Arthrocentesis is surgical puncture of a joint to remove fluid. This may be done for therapeutic and/or diagnostic purposes. -centesis is a suffix meaning surgical puncture. Arthrodesis is a binding or stabilization of a joint by operative means. -desis is a suffix meaning binding. Arthroplasty is surgical repair of a joint. -plasty is a suffix meaning surgical repair. Meniscectomy is the removal of a meniscus in a joint. The usual site of a meniscus removal is the knee. A syndesmoplasty is surgical repair of a ligament. Tenomyoplasty is the surgical repair of a tendon and a muscle. Ten/o is a combining form for a tendon, and my/o is a combining form for a muscle.

The musculoskeletal system is a complex set of bones, muscles, tendons, and ligaments that allow us to function. Our goal is to be able to accurately document, communicate, and understand the many terms and definitions that relate to this system.

CHAPTER 5

Digestive

The digestive system (gastrointestinal system) in the simplest of terms is one long tube that runs from the mouth to the anus. This system is commonly referred to as the GI tract. This tube is about 30 feet in length in adults and has three primary functions: digestion, absorption, and elimination. Digestion is defined as the process in which food is changed in the mouth, stomach, and intestines by chemical, mechanical, and physical action. This allows the body to break down the food so it is absorbed. Absorption is defined as when nutrient material is taken into the bloodstream and travels to all cells of the body. Elimination is defined as the process where the solid waste products of digestion are excreted.

- The functions of the GI system include: 1. ingestion: the intake of food; 2. digestion: the physical and chemical breakdown of food; 3. absorption: the extraction of nutrients; and 4. elimination: the excretion of waste products.
- The medical term for the waste products of the GI system is *feces*. The process of releasing feces from the body is defecation. You may have heard the abbreviation BM referring to bowel movements. This is another term for feces.
- Gastroenterologist treats disorders of the digestive system, exodontists remove teeth, periodontists treat the gums, pedodondists are children's dentists, proctologists treat disorders of the anus and rectum.
- The oral cavity is responsible for the function of mastication (chewing) and deglutition (swallowing). The combining forms stom/o and stomat/o refer literally to a mouth or an opening.
- The incisors and cuspids are the teeth that are located in the anterior (front) of the mouth, while the bicuspids and molars are located in the posterior (back) of the mouth. The incisors and cuspids serve to tear and break apart food, while the bicuspids and molars function to chew (masticate) the food. The word part cusp/o refers to point. In this case, the cuspids have a single "point," while the bicuspids have two.

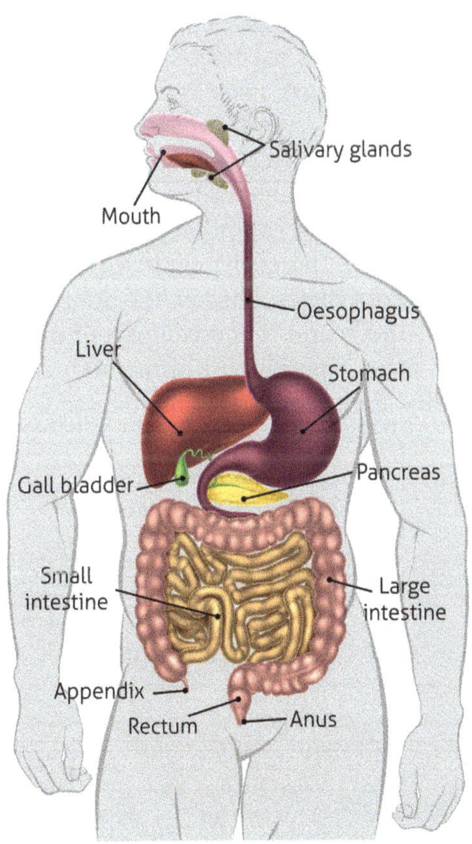

© Christos Georghiou/Shutterstock.com

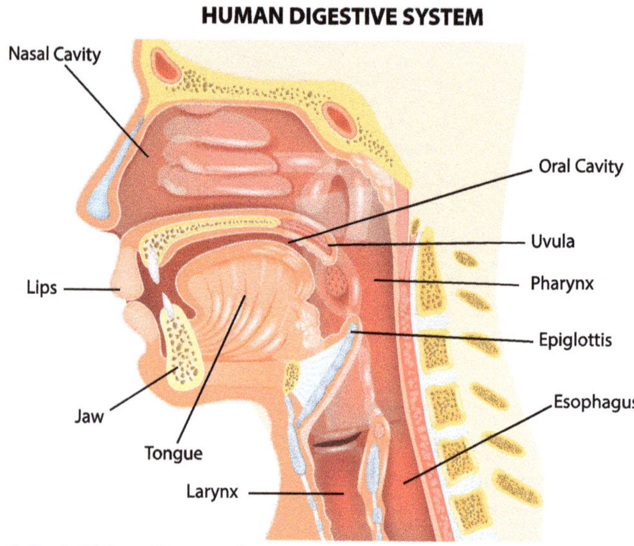

- The term *uvula* comes from the Latin meaning literally "little grape." Perhaps the uvula does appear to be a small grape that hangs from the back of the soft palate, but our best meaning for uvul/o is the uvula.
- There are three salivary glands, each named for its location. The parotid gland is near (par-) the ear (ot/o), the sublinugal gland is under (sub-) the tongue (lingu/o), and the submandibular gland is under (sub-) the lower jawbone (mandibul/o).

After chewing and swallowing a mouthful of food, the food enters the pharynx (the throat). There are three sections of the throat: the first, the nasopharynx, is behind the nasal cavity; the second, the oropharynx, is behind the oral cavity; and the third, the hypopharynx, is the area of the throat that is below the oropharynx. Another term that is sometimes used for the hypopharynx is the laryngopharynx because it is near the larynx, the voice box.

The esophagus is a muscular tube, about 12 inches long, that extends from the throat to the stomach. The masticated lump of food that is swallowed is termed the *bolus.* If you've ever swallowed a piece of meat that is too big, you may have experienced the peristaltic motion of this bolus being pushed toward the stomach.

The sphincter muscle (a round muscle) that opens and closes to allow the food into the stomach is called the lower esophageal sphincter, abbreviated LES, the cardiac sphincter, and the gastroesophageal sphincter. The first and last terms are understandable, but what about "cardiac sphincter"? It gets its name from its proximity to the heart.

From the esophagus, the bolus enters the stomach in the area of the cardia (again, because it is near the heart). The main part of the stomach is called the body, or corporis. The gastric fundus is the most superior part of the body of the stomach. The end of the stomach where the food exits is called the pylorus (also referred to as the gastric antrum).

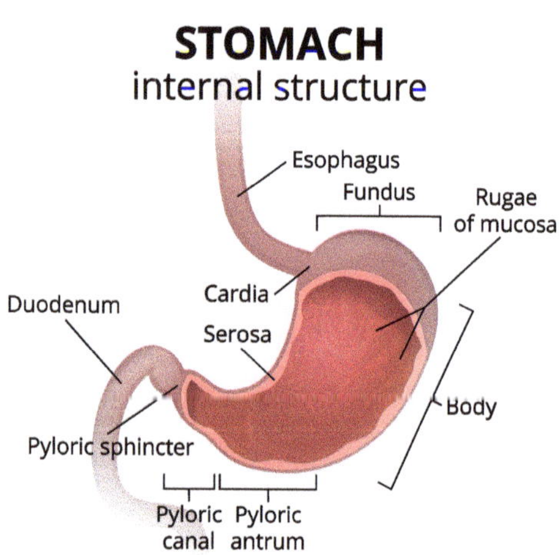

Digestion continues its chemical breakdown of the masticated food by mixing it with gastric juices and hydrochloric acid. The mixture of the food with the gastric juices and acid is termed *chyme.* The stomach is lined with ridges called *rugae* (s. ruga).

- The main function of the small intestines is the absorption of nutrients from the chyme. The structure of the intestines is a series of folds (plicae) that contain thousands of tiny projections termed villi (s. villus), which contain blood capillaries that absorb the products of carbohydrate and protein digestion. The three sections of the small intestines in order are the duodenum, the jejunum, and the ileum. The large intestines, also called the bowels, are much shorter in length than the small intestines, about 5 feet. The adjective "large" comes from the diameter. The main function of the large intestines is the elimination of waste products and the synthesis of vitamins. The waste that is in the intestines at this point is no longer chyme, but is now called feces.

Liver, Gallbladder, Pancreas and Bile Passage

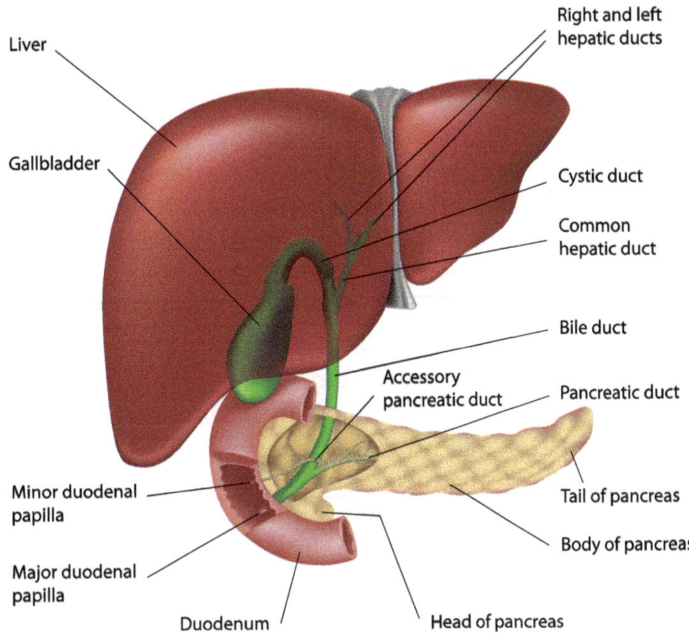

The first part of the large intestine is the cecum. The sphincter between the ileum and the cecum is the ileocecal sphincter. The vermiform appendix hangs from the cecum. Although it has no function in the digestive system, it may have a function in the lymphatic system. From the cecum, the feces travel up the ascending colon, across the transverse colon, down the descending colon, through the sigmoid colon (sigmoid—literally means "S" like), and finally through the rectum and out the anal sphincter.

The liver is composed of two lobes and is located mostly in the upper right quadrant of the abdominal cavity. Liver produces bile that emulsifies (breaks down) fats. Bile is composed of bilirubin, the waste product formed by the normal breakdown of hemoglobin in red blood cells at the end of their life spans, and cholesterol, a fatty substance found only in animal tissues. The gallbladder is a small sac that is found on the underside of the right lobe of the liver. Its function is to store bile until needed in digestion. When fatty food enters the duodenum, cholecystokinin is secreted, which causes the gallbladder to contract and release bile into the cystic duct. Note that -kinin is a suffix for a substance that moves, making cholecystokinin, a substance that moves the gallbladder. From the cystic duct, it travels to the common bile duct and then on to the duodenum. The pancreas is located in the upper left quadrant behind the stomach. It is involved in the digestion of carbohydrates, proteins, and fats (lipids). Pancreatic involvement in the digestive function is considered exocrine (meaning to secrete out) because it is through a duct. Later we will discuss the endocrine function of the pancreas, where it secretes within the bloodstream (endocrine).

Upper and Lower GI Complaints

Dyspepsia is the medical term for indigestion. Dys- means bad, difficult, or painful and the suffix -pepsia stands for digestion. Eructation is a medical term for the expulsion of air from the stomach through the mouth. You may recognize this as belching or burping. If air is swallowed, either intentionally or unintentionally, while eating, the term is aerophagia (aer/o = air + -phagia = condition of eating/swallowing). Halitosis is literally an abnormal condition of the breath, although it is generally considered to be bad breath. Pyrosis is a medical term for heartburn. It comes from the combining form for fire (pyr/o) and the suffix (-osis) for abnormal condition. Hiccups are involuntary contractions of the diaphragm, followed by a rapid closure of the glottis (the area where the vocal cords are located). Hiccup can also be spelled hiccough. Another synonym is singultus. Nausea is a sensation that accompanies the urge to vomit. Its word derivation is related to the word *nautical*, having to do with the ocean; hence, the term for sea sickness. Regurgitation is the return of swallowed food to the mouth. It can also be used to describe any backward flow (e.g., mitral regurgitation in the cardiovascular system) elsewhere in the body. Vomiting is the forceful or involuntary emptying of the contents of the stomach through the mouth. The medical term for the product of vomiting is vomitus, also called emesis. Emesis is also used as a medical suffix. Hematemesis is the vomiting of blood (hemat/o = blood). A common abbreviation used in describing patient complaints is N&V, which stands for nausea and vomiting. Constipation is infrequent, incomplete, or delayed bowel movements (BM). Obstipation is extreme constipation or intestinal obstruction. Diarrhea is an abnormal discharge of watery, semisolid stools. Flatus is gas passed through the anus. Hematochezia is bright red (frank) blood in the stools (-chezia = condition of stools). Melena is black, tarry stools caused by the presence of partially digested blood (melan/o = black, dark). Irritable bowel syndrome is a group of symptoms marked by diarrhea/gas/constipation resulting from stress with no underlying disease.

A cleft palate is a failure of the roof of the mouth to close during embryonic development, resulting in an opening of the roof of the mouth.

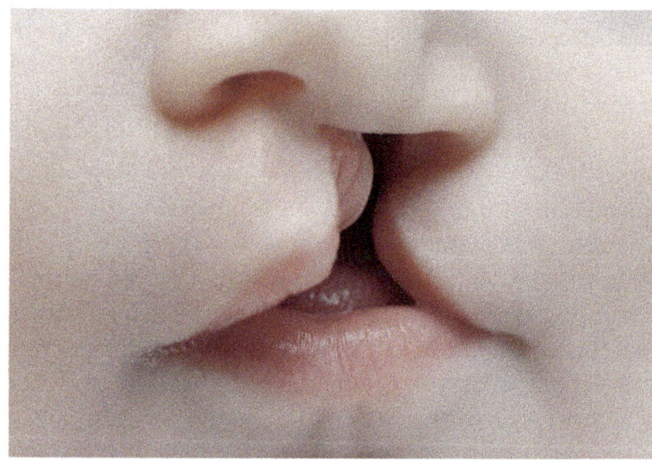

© malost/Shutterstock.com

Esophageal atresia (a- = without + = tresia condition of an opening) is a condition of the esophagus ending in a blind pouch and therefore lacking an opening into the stomach.

Hirschsprung disease is a congenital absence of normal nervous function in part of the colon, resulting in an absence of peristaltic movement, accumulation of feces, and an enlarged colon. A synonym is congenital megacolon (mega- = large).

Pyloric stenosis is a narrowing of the pyloric sphincter muscle, which prevents partially digested food from passing into the duodenum. Aphthous stomatitis is an inflammation of the mouth with the presence of small ulcers (aphth/o = ulceration). These erosions appear on the mucous membranes of the mouth. A synonym is canker sores. Cheilitis is an inflammation of the lips, while cheilosis is an abnormal condition of the lips that is present with riboflavin deficiency. Malocclusion (mal- + -occlusion) is misalignment of the upper and lower teeth. Dental caries are commonly known as cavities. The caries are caused by an interaction between food and bacteria in the mouth. Dental plaque is a film of material that coats the teeth and may lead to decay if not removed. Achalasia (a- + -chalasia) is a condition of being without relaxation. It is an impairment of the normal peristaltic movement of the esophagus, along with an inability of the lower esophageal sphincter to relax and allow a bolus of food into the stomach. Synonyms for achalasia include esophageal aperistalsis (again, notice the prefix a- meaning no, not, without), megaesophagus (mega- meaning large), and cardiospasm, meaning an involuntary contraction (-spasm) of the cardiac sphincter (cardi/o)—*not the heart!* Dysphagia means difficulty with swallowing. One of our acronyms, GERD, signifies a return of the contents of the stomach to the esophagus because of the LES's inability to remain contracted. It is the opposite of achalasia! Symptoms may include pyrosis (heart burn) and regurgitation. Another disorder, Barrett esophagus, is a condition that is often associated with the chronic irritation of the esophagus by GERD. This disorder is associated with an increased risk of cancer.

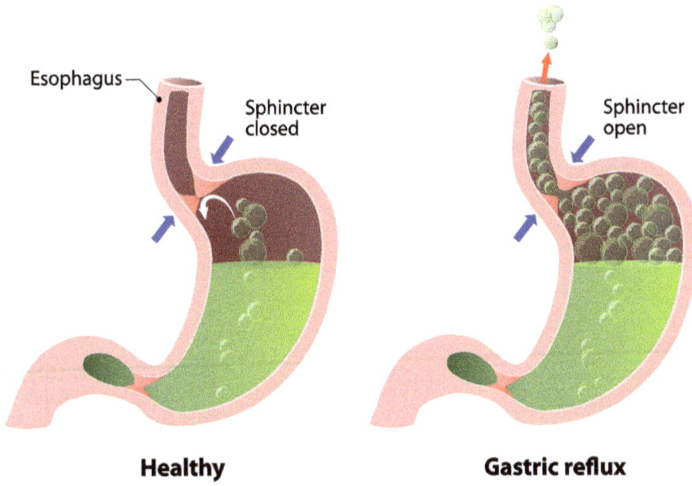

© Designua/Shutterstock.com

- Gastralgia is pain of the stomach, stomach pain, or a stomachache. Gastritis is an inflammation of the stomach. Peptic ulcer disease gets its name *peptic* meaning pertaining to digestion. Therefore, this is a type of erosion of the mucosal lining of the GI system. It occurs most often in the stomach or duodenum. Appendicitis (appendic/o + -itis) is an inflammation of the appendix.

Peritonitis is an inflammation of the peritoneum, the lining of the abdominal cavity. It can occur if the appendicitis is not treated and the appendix bursts.

Colitis is an inflammation of the colon. Crohn disease is an inflammation of the ileum or the colon that is of idiopathic origin. Also called regional or granulomatous enteritis.

Inflammatory bowel disease (IBD) is a chronic inflammation of the lining of the intestine characterized by bleeding and diarrhea. Ulcerative colitis is a chronic inflammation of the colon and rectum manifested by bouts of profuse watery diarrhea. Diverticula are pouches in the lining of the colon. Diverticulosis is the abnormal condition of the presence of these pouches. Diverticulitis is an inflammation of the diverticula. A fistula is an abnormal opening between organs (internal) or to the outside of the body (external). This occurs as the result of a disease process, not a surgical intervention. A fistula is an abnormal opening between organs (internal) or to the outside of the body (external). This occurs as the result of a disease process, not a surgical intervention. Cirrhosis is a chronic degenerative disease of the liver, usually associated with alcohol abuse. Cirrh/o means an orange-yellow color, referring to the accompanying jaundice. Hepatitis is an inflammation of the liver that is caused by a variety of viruses.

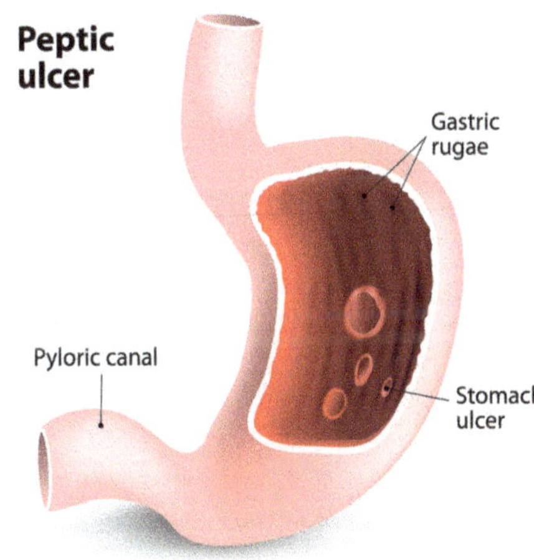

© Designua/Shutterstock.com

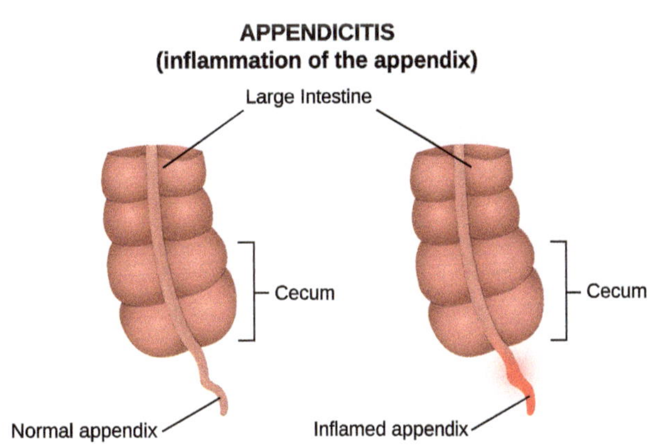

© Marochkina Anastasiia/Shutterstock.com

Strangulated Hernia

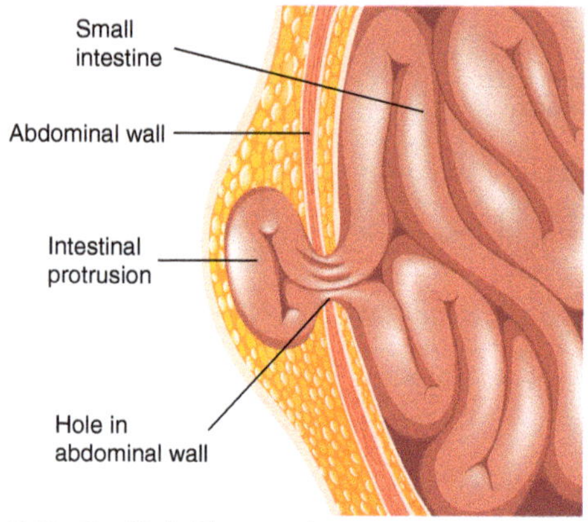

Hepatitis A is transmitted through direct contact with fecally contaminated food or water.

Hepatitis B is transmitted through contaminated blood or sexual contact.

Hepatitis C is transmitted through blood transfusions, percutaneous inoculation, or through the sharing of infected needles.

Jaundice is a yellowing of the skin and sclerae.

Pancreatitis is an inflammation of the pancreas.

A femoral hernia is the protrusion of a loop of intestine through the femoral canal into the groin. It is the same as a crural hernia.

A hiatal hernia is a protrusion of part of the stomach through the diaphragm. It is also called a diaphragmatic hernia or a diaphragmatocele. (-cele meaning herniation or protrusion).

An inguinal hernia is a protrusion of a loop of bowel through the inguinal canal.

An umbilical hernia is a protrusion of the intestine and omentum (a fold of the peritoneum) through the abdominal wall. It is also called an omphalocele (omphal/o means umbilicus).

An incarcerated hernia occurs when a loop of bowel becomes occluded (blocked or closed) so that solids cannot pass. It is also called an irreducible hernia.

Hemorrhoid

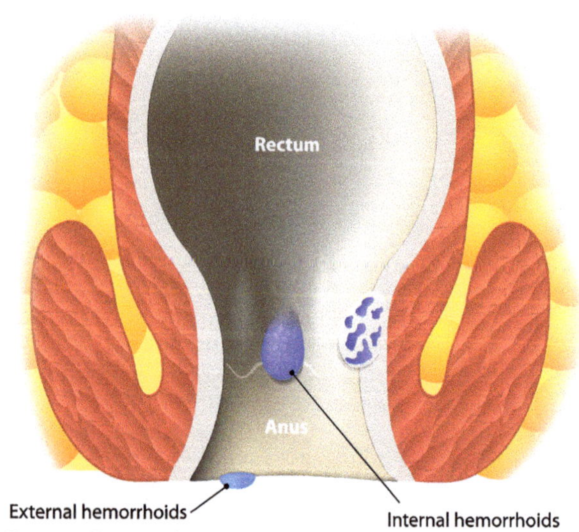

Strangulation is the constriction (narrowing) of a tubular structure. A strangulated hernia is one in which the blood flow is shut off.

A hemorrhoidectomy would be the removal of hemorrhoids.

A herniorrhaphy is literally a suturing of a hernia, or a hernia repair.

Laparoscopic surgery is surgery through several small incisions in the abdominal wall using a laparoscope. A cholecystectomy is the removal of the gallbladder.

The gastrointestinal system is a complex system that allows our body to process nutrients. In order for our body to maintain its optimal performance, we must put the right things in it in the right amount for our entire body system to function properly. The GI tract is paramount in our body's ability to do those things.

CHAPTER 6

Blood and Lymph

Blood is one of the two main fluids in the body. It is circulated throughout the body with the heart functioning as the pump. Lymph is the other main fluid in the body and is circulated throughout the body in complex system of vessels. Blood is the fluid consisting of formed elements and plasma. We will detail the specifics about blood in this chapter. The functions of this system are to transport, regulate, protect, and defend. The blood, lymphatic, and immune systems are three integrated systems that help the body maintain homeostasis, a steady state. The functions of the blood are to provide transportation of gases (oxygen and carbon dioxide), hormones, nutrients, salts, and cells that defend the body; to regulate the body's fluid and electrolyte balance, acid–base balance, and body temperature; to protect the body from infection; and to protect the body from loss of blood through the action of clotting. Hematology is the study, diagnosis, and treatment of diseases of blood and blood-forming organs. The specialist in this field is a hematologist. The lymphatic system is responsible for cleaning the cellular environment, returning proteins and tissue fluids to the blood (as a means of drainage), providing a pathway for the absorption of fats and fat-soluble vitamins into the bloodstream, and defending the body against disease. The immune system is responsible for defending the body against disease via the immune response. The combining form immun/o means safety or protection. Immunology is the study, diagnosis, and treatment of diseases that affect the body's ability to defend itself. The specialist in this field is an immunologist. Immunology is the study, diagnosis, and treatment of diseases that affect the body's ability to defend itself. The specialist in this field is an immunologist.

The blood and lymph flow through separate but interdependent channels. Both are systems composed of vessels and the liquids that flow through them. The immune system, a complex system of levels of protection for the body, includes both blood and lymphatic cells.

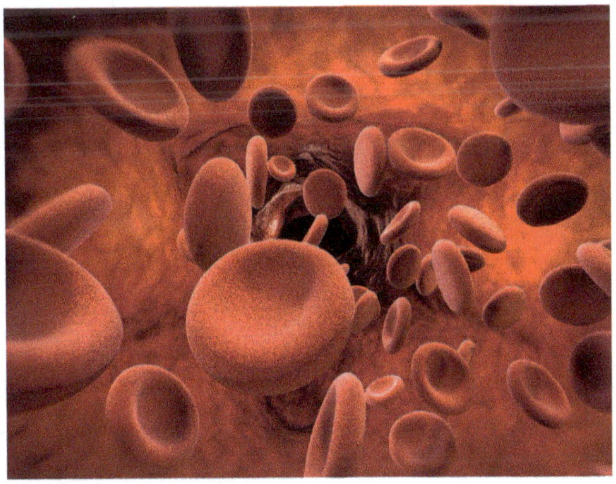

Hematopoiesis (hemat/o = blood + -poiesis = formation) is the process of the formation of blood. All blood cells originate from a single type of cell called a stem cell. The liquid tissue of blood is composed of a solid portion that is made up of cells and a liquid portion called the plasma. The cells make up approximately 45% of the total blood volume, and plasma is the other 55%. These numbers vary slightly

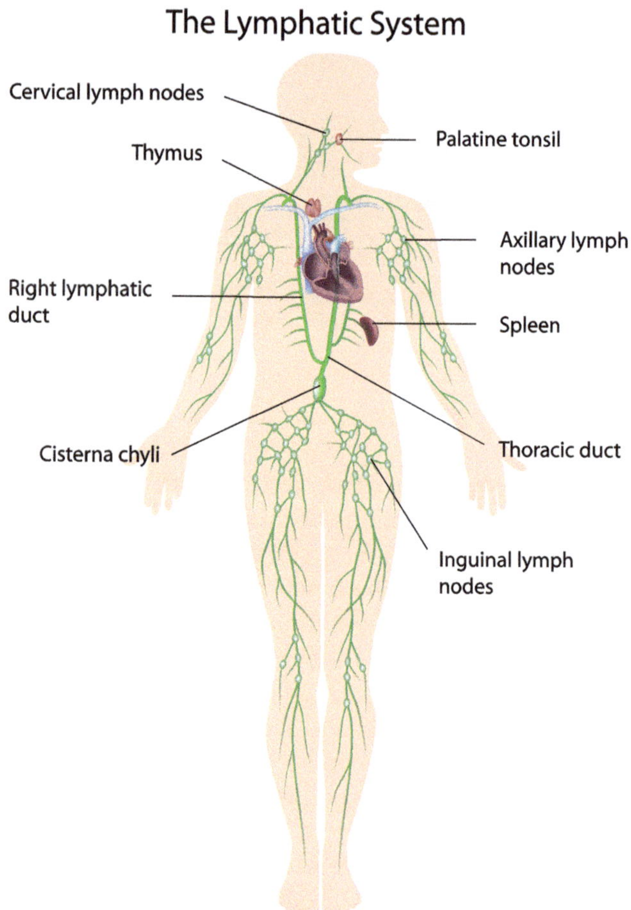

depending on an individual's sex, but are important in the measurement of a hematocrit, a test that will be discussed in the diagnostic terms section. The three types of blood cells are red blood cells called erythrocytes, white blood cells called leukocytes, and clotting cells called thrombocytes or platelets. To have an idea of their relative numbers, in a milliliter of blood there are 4.2–5.8 million red blood cells, 5000–9000 white blood cells, and 250,000–400,000 thrombocytes. Blood itself accounts for about 8% of the total body volume and the average volume of blood is about 10.5 pts or 5 L (think of your favorite soda) in a 150-lb (or 68-kg) person.

Aside from the function of transporting oxygen and carbon dioxide throughout the body, the blood must also carry a protein–iron pigment called hemoglobin. Red blood cells are formed in the bone marrow as a result of stimulation by a hormone in the kidneys called erythropoietin (erythr/o = red [blood cell] + -poietin = forming substance). The life cycle of a red blood cell is about 4 months or 120 days, after which time it decomposes into hemosiderin (hem/o + siderin = iron substance), which is an iron pigment resulting from hemolysis (-lysis = breaking down). Aside from the hemosiderin, bilirubin is also a by-product of the decomposition. The iron is stored in the liver for recycling and the bile pigments are excreted by the liver. The morphology of blood cells is important (morph/o = shape). Normal blood cells have a biconcave, disk-like shape, which moves easily throughout the vessels. In some disorders, such as sickle cell anemia, the shape of the cells is changed, which results in dysfunction and disease.

Leukocytes, in general, protect the body from invasion by pathogens. There are two main types of these white blood cells.

The first type, granulocytes (also called polymorphonucleocytes), are named for the small grains within the cytoplasm and mutlilobed nuclei. Granul/o = little grain. Poly- means many + morph/o = shape + nucle/o = nucleus + -cyte = cell. The two names are used interchangeably and you should be familiar with both. There are three types of granulocytes:

Eosinophils (eosin/o = rosy-colored + -phil = attraction) are cells that absorb a rosy-colored acidic dye, which causes them to have a reddish color. An increase in eosinophils is usually the body's response to defending itself against allergens.

Neutrophils (neutr/o = neutral) are cells that are neither acidic nor alkaline, and they stain a lavender/purplish color. An increase in neutrophils is normal when the body is combating

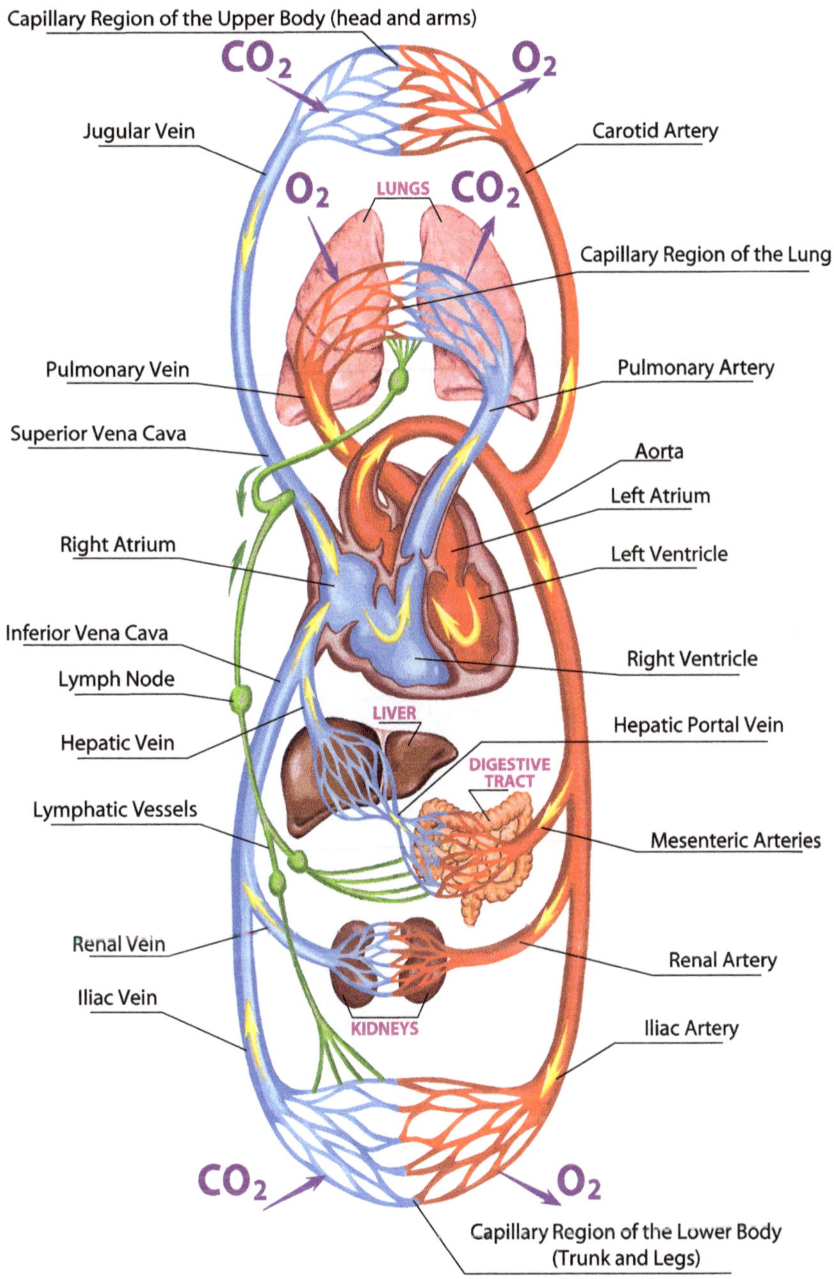

bacteria in pyogenic (py/o = pus + -genic pertaining to producing) infections. The cells perform the function of phagocytosis (phag/o = eat, swallow), where they consume the "enemies" and remove the debris from the battlefield.

Basophils (bas/o = base) are cells that absorb a basic dye and stain a bluish color. They release histamine in response to inflammation and heparin to heal damaged tissue.

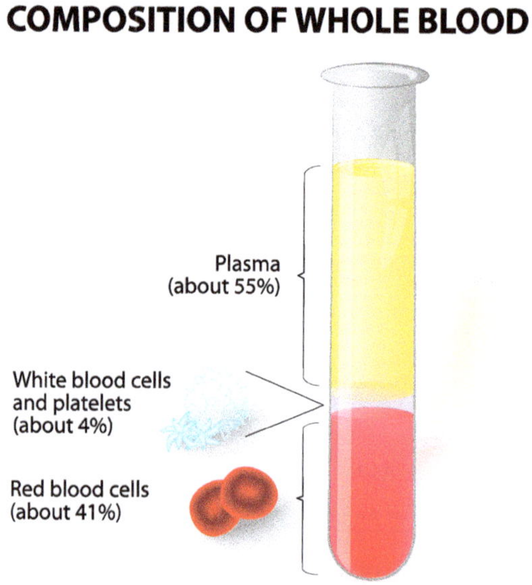

© Designua/Shutterstock.com

Agranulocytes are the second type of leukocyte. Notice that an a- has been added denoting the absence of the small grains in the appearance of these cells. They, too, have another name: mononuclear leukocytes, because their nuclei have only one nucleus. Although these cells originate in the bone marrow, they mature only after entering the lymphatic system.

There are two types: monocytes and lymphocytes. Monocytes are named for their single, large nucleus. These cells are transformed into cells call macrophages (macro- = large + -phage = eat, swallow), which eat pathogens and are called out for severe infections. Lymphocytes are cells that are important in the immune response, meaning that they recognize or remember dangerous foreign substances and manufacture a substance to neutralize them. The foreign substances are termed *antigens* and the neutralizing substances are called *antibodies*.

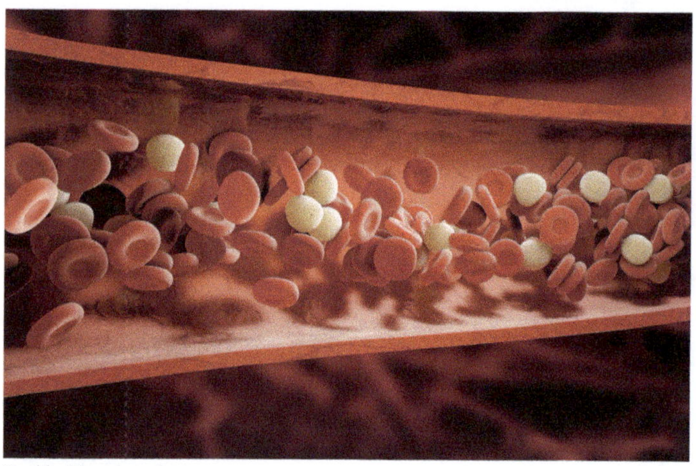

© adike/Shutterstock.com

Thrombocytes (platelets) have a round or oval shape and the name platelet comes from their appearance as little plates. These cells aid in the coagulation (clotting) of the blood, which is the process of changing a liquid to a solid. The process of coagulation begins with agglutination, which is a clumping of the cells. The cells release a substance called Factor X (formerly called thrombokinase),

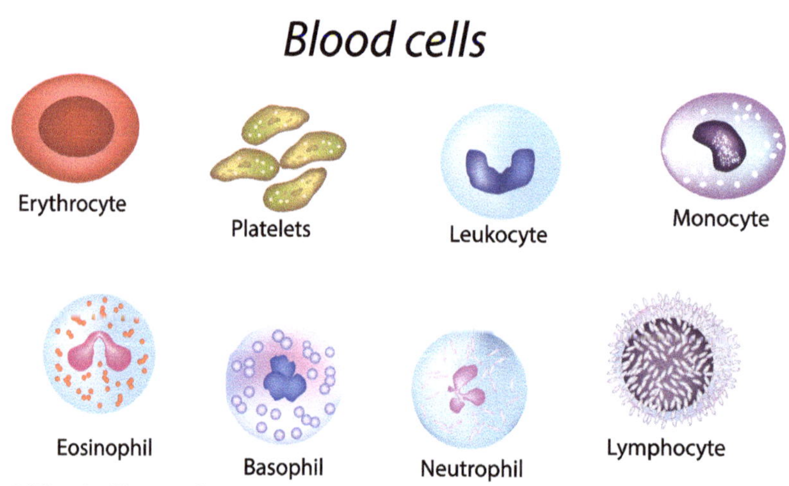

© Timonina/Shutterstock.com

which, in the presence of calcium, reacts with the blood protein, prothrombin. Prothrombin then forms thrombin. Thrombin converts to form another blood protein, fibrinogen. Fibrinogen is then converted to fibrin, which eventually forms a mesh-like fibrin clot. Hemostasis (hem/o = blood + -stasis = stopping, controlling), or the control of blood flow, is then achieved.

Plasma, the liquid portion of blood, is composed of:

- Water.
- Inorganic substances (calcium, potassium, sodium).
- Organic substances (glucose, amino acids, fats, cholesterol, hormones).
- Waste products (urea, uric acid, ammonia, creatinine).
- Plasma proteins (serum albumin and serum globulin) and clotting proteins (fibrinogen and prothrombin).

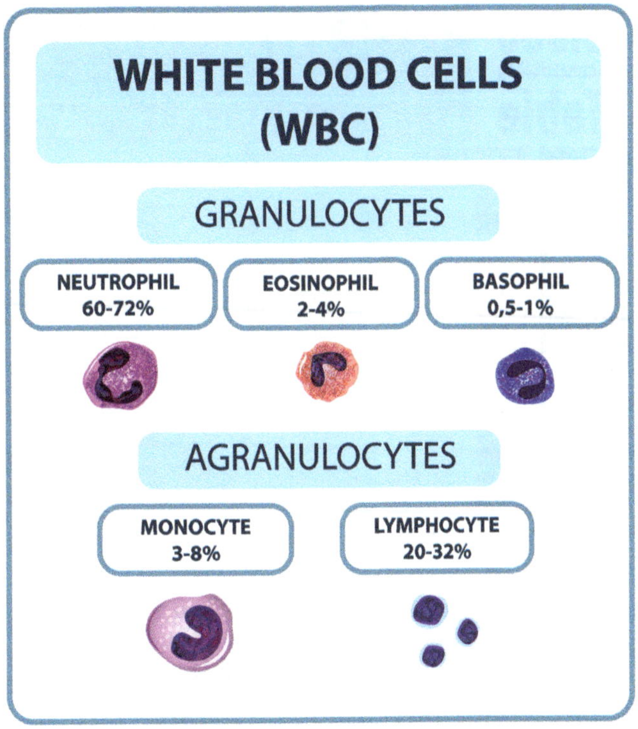

© JuliaL/Shutterstock.com

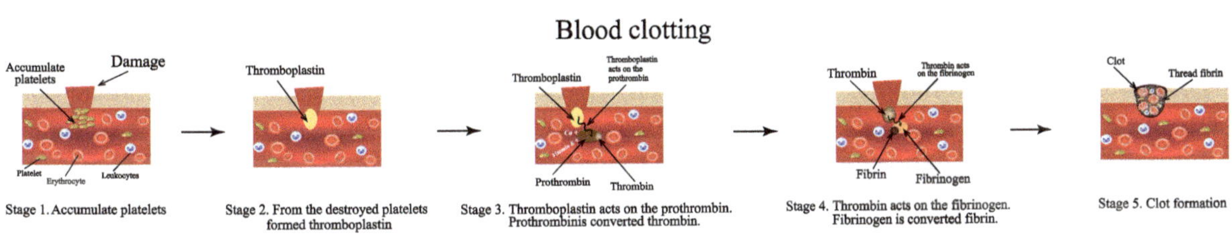

© Timonina/Shutterstock.com

Serum is plasma minus the clotting proteins (fibrinogen and prothrombin). Serology is the branch of laboratory medicine that studies blood serum for evidence of infection by evaluating antigen–antibody reactions *in vitro (in living tissue)*.

Human blood is divided into four major blood groups. They are named A, B, AB, and O. The differences are due to antigens present on the surface of an individual's blood cells. Remember that antigens are substances that produce an immune reaction by their nature of being perceived as foreign to the body. Because of this recognition as "foreign," the body produces substances called antibodies to neutralize the "invader." In blood, the antigens are called agglutinogens [because they are substances that produce (gen) clumping substances (agglutin/o)] and the antibodies are called agglutinins.

Type A blood has A antigens, type B has type B antigens, type AB has type a and type B antigens, and type O has neither A nor B antigens.

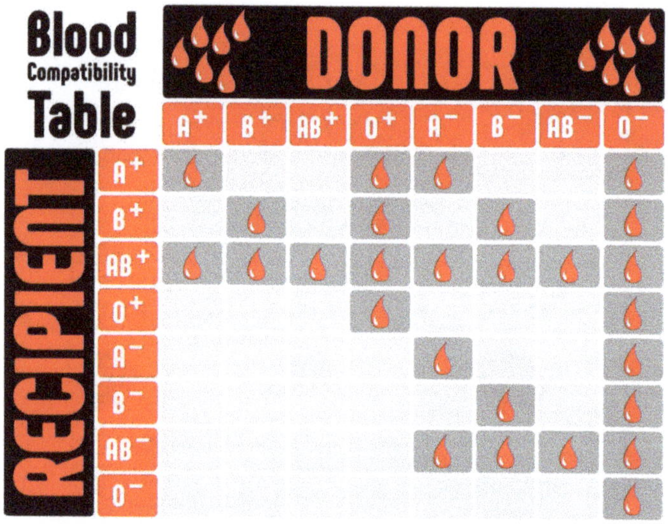

© udaix/Shutterstock.com

Therefore, if a type A individual is transfused with type B blood, the blood will agglutinate because type B blood is perceived as foreign. However, this same type A individual could be transfused with type O blood, because it has neither type A nor type B antigens.

Type O blood, therefore, is the universal donor, because it has no antigens that will cause a reaction with any of the blood types. Type AB, however, is referred to as a universal recipient, because it has both type A and type B antigens.

The Rh factor, another antigen, is important in pregnancy because a mother who is Rh− can develop antibodies to an Rh+ fetus in the first pregnancy and cause hemolysis (-lysis = destruction) of the fetus' blood in subsequent pregnancies.

The lymphatic system is composed of lymph, also called interstitial fluid, which is the fluid surrounding the cells; lymph vessels, which are small valvular structures; lymph glands (also called lymph nodes); and lymph organs (tonsils, adenoids, appendix, spleen, thymus gland, Peyer patches, and lymphoid tissue). Monocytes and lymphocytes pass out of the bloodstream and into the lymphatic fluid through the capillary walls in the spaces between cells in the body tissue. Monocytes change into macrophages, destroy pathogens, and collect debris from damaged cells. Lymphocytic function will be discussed with the immune system. Lymph moves in one direction (hence the valves in the lymph vessels) in order to prevent pathogens from flowing through the body. From the lymph vessels, the flow continues to the lymph gland and on to either the right lymphatic duct or the thoracic duct, both of which empty into the subclavian veins in the neck. Once back in the venous blood, the lymph is recycled through the body for another round. The system filters out the microorganisms as the lymph passes through its various systemic structures. The major lymph glands are the cervical (cervic/o = neck), axillary (axill/o = armpit), inguinal (inguin/o = groin), and mediastinal nodes.

The immune system is composed of organs, tissues, cells, and chemical messengers that interact to protect the body from external invaders and its own internally altered cells. Cytokines (cyt/o = cell + -kine = movement) are the chemical messengers that are secreted by cells of the immune system that direct immune cellular interaction. Lymphocytes secrete lymphokines and monocytes and macrophages secrete monokines. Interleukins (inter- = between = -leukin white substance) are a type of cytokine that sends messages "between" leukocytes to direct protective action. The levels of defense provided by the immune system are divided into a first line, which is a nonspecific immunity; a second line, which is another type of nonspecific immunity; and a third line of defense, which is a specific type of immunity.

The first line of defense includes three different methods of warding off pathogens, without having to recognize them. They are:

- Mechanical: the barrier of the intact skin, the sticky mucus on mucous membranes.
- Physical: coughing, sneezing, vomiting, diarrhea.
- Chemical: tears, saliva, perspiration.

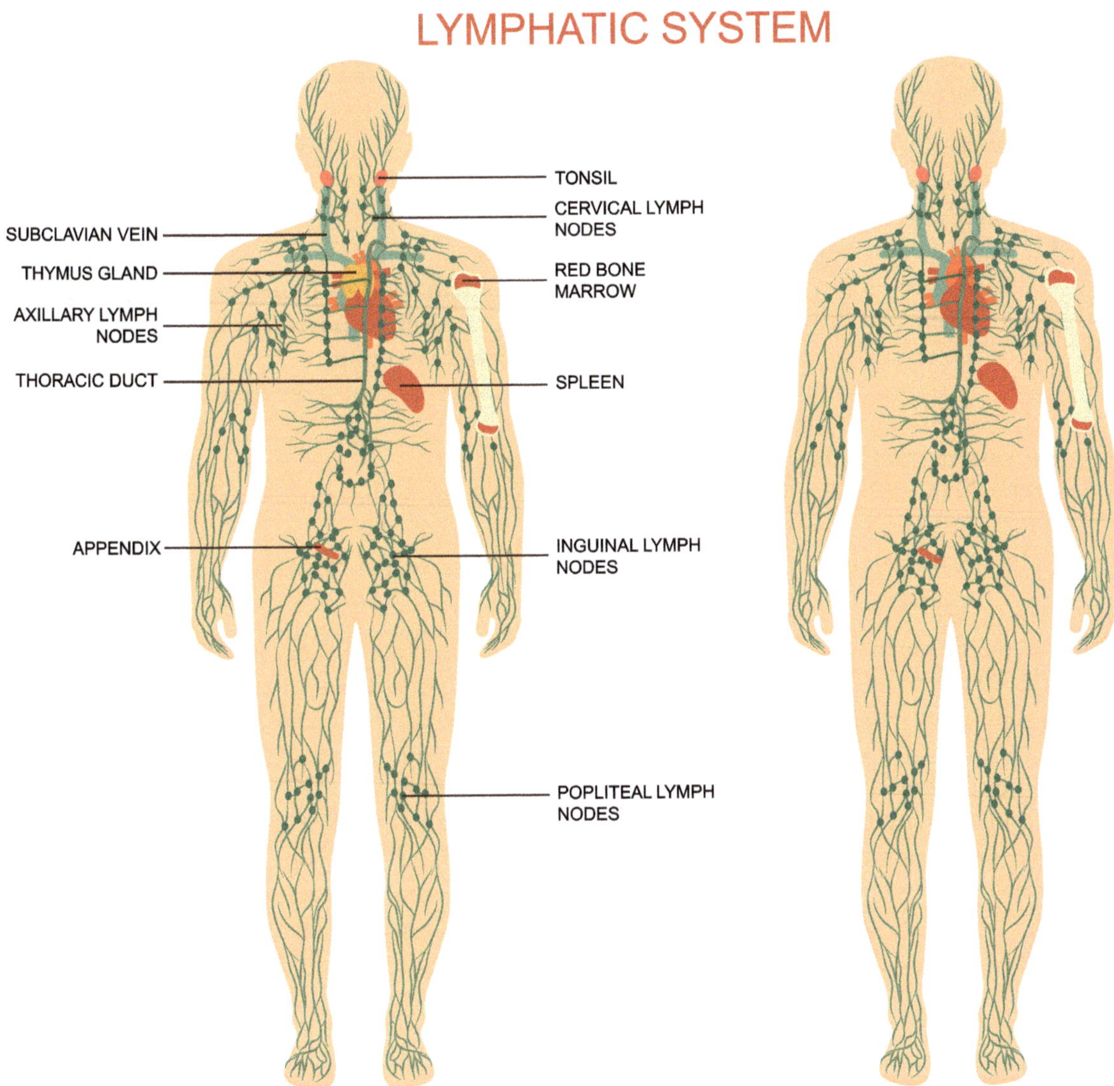

The second line of defense comes into play if the pathogens make it past the first line of defense. These include:

- Phagocytosis: the neutrophils and monocytes.
- Inflammation: heat, swelling, redness, and pain.
- Pyrexia: fever (pyr/o = fire).
- Protective proteins:
  - Interferon disrupts viral replication.
  - Complement proteins: inactive forms that are activated in the presence of bacteria to lyse (destroy) an organism.

Natural killer cells: a specific type of lymphocyte that acts nonspecifically to kill cells infected by certain viruses and cancer cells.

Specific immunity means that the immune response is tailored for a particular organism. The antibodies formed for the particular antigens are termed immunoglobulins. The recognition of the pathogen can be genetically determined or acquired.

- If genetically determined, individuals inherit the ability to resist certain diseases because of their species, race, sex, or individual genetics.
- Acquired forms of immunity are either active or passive.
    - Active acquired immunity
        - Natural immunity is the development of memory cells to protect an individual from a second exposure (because individuals were exposed to chicken pox and came down with it, they are then immune to another round).
        - Artificial immunity: vaccinations (immunizations) use a weakened form to enable the body to form antibodies.
    - Passive acquired immunity
        - Natural passive immunity is the passage of antibodies through the placenta or breast milk.
        - Artificial passive immunity is the use of Ig harvested from a donor who developed immunity against specific antigens.

The term anemia means (an- no, not, without + -emia—blood condition). Patients with anemia are not literally "without blood," they are just lacking a specific constituent of blood or may be deficient in the normal blood volume. An acute posthemorrhagic anemia is a red blood cell deficiency caused by blood loss. Chronic blood loss is long-term internal bleeding that may cause anemia. Sideropenia is a deficiency of iron in the blood (sider/o = iron + -penia = deficiency). This may be due to chronic blood loss, inadequate iron intake, or unspecified causes. It is a type of an iron deficiency anemia. Pernicious anemia is a progressive anemia that results from a lack of intrinisic factor essential for the absorption of vitamin B_{12}. B_{12} deficiency is an insufficient blood level of cobalamin, also called vitamin B_{12}, which is necessary for mature RBCs. It may be caused by inadequate dietary intake or by the absence of intrinsic factor, a substance necessary for B_{12} absorption. Folate deficiency is an anemia that results from a lack of folate from dietary, drug-induced, congenital, or other causes. Hypovolemia (vol/o = volume) is a deficiency of the volume of circulating blood.

Sickle cell anemia is an inherited anemia characterized by crescent-shaped RBCs. The change in morphology (morph/o = shape, form) causes the RBCs to block the small-diameter capillaries, which results in a decreased blood supply to the cells. A sickle cell crisis is an acute, painful exacerbation of sickle cell anemia. Use the diagrams to discuss how the morphology of sickle cells causes dysfunction.

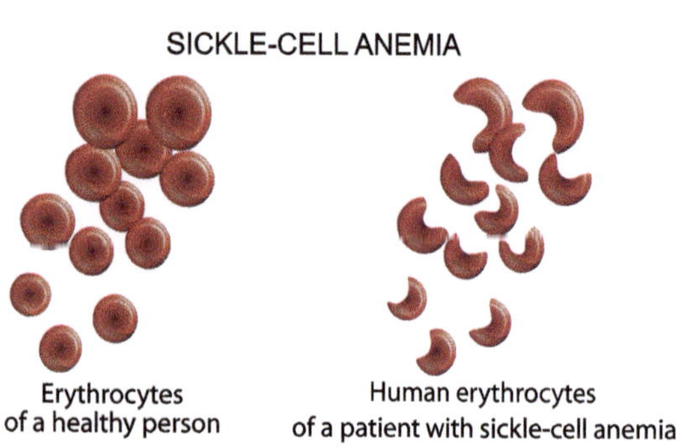

Approximately 8% of African-Americans carry the sickle cell gene, and 1 in 400 is affected with the disease. Sickle cell anemia is expressed only in individuals who inherit the gene from both parents. If only one gene is present, the patient is said to have the sickle cell trait.

Hemophilia is a group of inherited bleeding disorders characterized by a deficiency of one of the factors necessary for the coagulation of blood. The suffix -philia means a tendency; in this case, to bleed.

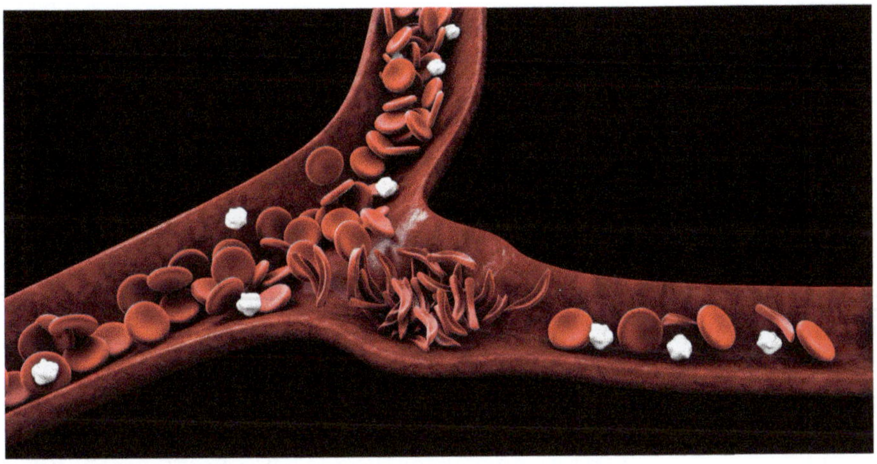

© Victor Josan/Shutterstock.com

Septicemia (sept/o = infection + -emia = blood condition) is a systemic infection in the blood caused by pathogens that have spread from elsewhere in the body. Septic shock is the result of low blood pressure caused by overwhelming infection. Organs fail and death may occur. Systemic inflammatory response syndrome is a type of septic shock characterized by an inflammatory state affecting the whole body. It may be caused by infection, trauma, ischemia, or inflammations. Edema is an abnormal accumulation of fluid in the interstitial spaces of tissues. Edema is one of those terms that can stand alone or as a suffix meaning swelling. Lymphedema is an accumulation of lymphatic fluid and resultant swelling caused by obstruction, removal, or hypoplasia of lymph vessels.

Acquired immunodeficiency syndrome (AIDS) is caused by the human immunodeficiency virus (HIV), transmitted through body fluids via sexual contact or intravenous exposure. HIV attacks the helper T cells, which causes a diminished immune response.

An allergy (also called a hypersensitivity) is an immune system's overreaction to irritants that are perceived as antigens. The substance that causes the irritation is termed an allergen.

Anaphylaxis is an extreme form of allergic response in which the patient suffers severe decreased blood pressure and constriction of the airways. The name for the condition comes from the original thought that this was a lack of protection (ana- without + -phylaxis = protection), not an overreaction of the body to the perceived threat.

An immediate allergy is a hypersensitivity caused by IgE. Examples are grass and tree pollens.

A delayed allergy is caused by activated T cells that respond to an exposure of the skin to a chemical irritant up to 2 days later. An example would be poison ivy. The resulting rash is called contact dermatitis.

There are several tests that physicians use to analyze our blood. AIDS tests, such as ELISA and the Western blot test, are done to detect the presence of HIV types 1 and 2. Allergy testing is a series of tests involving a patch, scratch, or intradermal injection of an attenuated amount of an allergen to test for hypersensitivity. A basic metabolic panel is a group of blood tests to measure calcium glucose, electrolytes such as sodium, potassium, chloride, creatinine, and blood urea nitrogen. Blood cultures are blood samples that are submitted to propagate microorganisms that may be present. Cultures may be indicated for bacteremia (bacteria in the blood) or septicemia (an infection in the blood) or to discover other pathogens such as fungi, viruses, or parasites. A complete blood cell count (CBC) is a set of 12 tests, including RBC (red blood cell count), WBC (white blood cell count), Hb (hemoglobin), Hct/PCV (hematocrit/packed-cell volume), and diff (WBC differential). A comprehensive metabolic panel (CMP) is a set of 14 blood tests that add protein and liver function tests to the BMP. Glucose is also measured by a different method than in the basic panel. A Coombs antiglobulin test is a blood test to diagnose hemolytic disease of the newborn (HDN), acquired hemolytic anemia, or a transfusion reaction. A white blood cell count is the measurement of the number of leukocytes in the blood. An increase may indicate the presence of an infection; a decrease may be caused by radiation or chemotherapy.

A bone marrow transplant is the removal of healthy bone marrow from either the patient or a donor for later transplantation. An autologous transplant (auto- means self) is bone marrow tissue taken from the patient before treatment to be reintroduced later to form healthy blood cells. A homologous transplant (homo- means same) is the transplantation of healthy bone marrow from a donor to a recipient to stimulate the formation of new blood cells.

An adenoidectomy is the removal of the pharyngeal tonsils (the adenoids). Biopsies of lymphatic structures are removal of the lymph nodes or lymphatic tissue as a means of diagnosis and treatment. A lymphadenectomy is the removal of a lymph node (the same as a lymph gland). A splenectomy is the removal of the spleen.

Here are a few medications that have a direct effect on our blood. Anticoagulants are drugs that prevent or delay the coagulation of blood and the formation of thrombi (blood clots). Examples include heparin, warfarin (Coumadin), enoxaparin (Lovenox), anisindione (Miradon), and lepirudin (Refludan).

Antiplatelets inhibit the function of platelets or destroy them. Examples include aspirin, clopidogrel (Plavix), dipyridamole (Persantine), ticlopidine (Ticlid), and abciximab (ReoPro).

Blood flow modifiers are drugs that promote blood flow by keeping platelets from clumping or decreasing blood viscosity. Examples include the prescription medications cilostazol (Pletal) and pentoxifylline (Trental) and the herbal product ginkgo biloba.

Colony-stimulating factors (CSFs) are agents that stimulate the production of white blood cells in the bone marrow. The two kinds are granulocyte CSF (G-CSF) and granulocyte-macrophage CSF (GM-CSF). Available synthetic agents of each type are filgrastim (Neupogen) and sargramostim (Leukine), respectively.

Erythropoietic agents are growth factors that increase the production of RBCs by stimulating erythropoiesis. Two available agents are epoetin-alfa (Epogen, Procrit) and darbepoetin-alfa (Aranesp).

Hematinics are drugs that increase the number of erythrocytes and/or hemoglobin concentration in the erythrocytes usually to treat iron-deficiency anemia. Examples are iron supplements and B-complex vitamins.

Hematopoietic agents are agents that stimulate blood cell production. Subdivisions of this class include colony-stimulating factors, erythropoietic agents, and thrombopoietic factors.

Hemostatics are drugs that help stop the flow of blood (-static = controlling the flow of blood). Examples include aminocaproic acid (Amicar) and tranexamic acid (Cyklokapron).

Thrombopoietic factors are agents that stimulate the production of thrombocytes or platelets. Oprelvekin (Neumega) is an available agent.

Antihistamines are drugs that block histamine receptors to manage allergy symptoms. Examples include clemastine (Tavist), diphenhydramine (Benadryl), loratadine (Claritin), and fexofenadine (Allegra).

Anti-IgE (immunoglobulin E) agents are monoclonal antibodies used to treat allergic asthma and allergic rhinitis. Omalizumab (Xolair) is the first available agent in this class.

Antineoplastics are drugs used to treat cancer by preventing the growth or promoting the destruction of neoplastic (tumor) cells. Numerous drugs, including methotrexate and rituximab (Rituxan), fall into this category.

Antiretrovirals are drugs that manage the replication of HIV and its progression into AIDS. Examples include zidovudine or AZT (Retrovir) and efavirenz (Sustiva).

Corticosteroids are drugs (also known as steroids) that suppress the immune system and reduce inflammation. Examples include fluticasone (Flovent, Flonase), hydrocortisone (Cortizone), and prednisone (Deltasone).

Cytotoxic agents are drugs used as immunosuppressants or antineoplastics in order to damage or destroy cells.

Immunosuppressants are drugs that reduce the immune response. Examples include azathioprine (Imuran), cyclophosphamide (Cytoxan), cyclosporine (Sandimmune), and tacrolimus (Prograf).

Leukotriene receptor antagonists are drugs that block leukotrienes to manage later stages of allergic reactions; they are used, in particular, to manage allergic asthma. The two agents in this class are montelukast (Singulair) and zafirlukast (Accolate).

Protease inhibitors are antiretroviral drugs used to treat HIV infections. By blocking the production of an essential enzyme called protease, these drugs keep the virus from replicating. Examples are indinavir (Crixivan), nelfinavir (Viracept), and saquinavir (Invirase).

Vaccines are substances administered to induce immunity or reduce the pathologic effects of a disease. Examples are the measles, mumps, rubella vaccine, and chicken pox vaccine.

CHAPTER 7

Cardiovascular

The cardiovascular system is a complex system of muscles, vessels, and electricity. Each has a very unique and specific purpose that allows our body to get oxygen to our cells and a mechanism for us to release carbon dioxide.

The function of the cardiovascular (cardi/o + vascul/o + -ar) system is to provide a means of transportation for a variety of substances to and from the cells of the body. The heart acts as a pump, while the vessels act as pipes to deliver the transportation medium, the blood, to the cells. The substances that need to be delivered are oxygen, nutrients, water, body salts, and hormones. The primary substance that needs to be hauled away is carbon dioxide. You may have heard an alternate term, the circulatory system, used to name this system. The diagnosis, treatment, and prevention of disorders of the heart are the discipline of cardiology. The specialist in this area is a cardiologist.

Notice that the circulation can be divided into two main areas: pulmonary (pulmon/o = lung + -ary = pertaining to) circulation and systemic (system/o = system + ic = pertaining to) circulation. Pulmonary circulation begins with the right side of the heart (notice that the blood is deoxygenated) where the blood is pushed out to the lungs to offload the carbon dioxide and pick up oxygen. Now oxygenated, the blood travels back to the left side of the heart where it is pumped out to begin its route through the systemic circulation. Note that pulmonary circulation is about the exchange of oxygen and carbon dioxide with the cells of the lungs. Systemic circulation describes the exchange of gases and substances between the blood and the cells of the body. The blood is pumped out of the left side of the heart through the aorta (the largest artery of the body) to a system of arteries that divide into smaller arterioles that end in tiny capillaries. The capillaries of the body tissues are the sites of exchange between the cells' fluids and the plasma of the circulatory system. The journey then begins back to the heart through tiny veins called venules, then larger veins, and finally the two largest veins of the body, the inferior and superior venae cavae.

Arteries are thick and muscular, necessary properties to withstand the force of the heartbeat, while veins are thinner and have one-way valves that prevent the backflow of blood. Capillaries are tiny and thin enough to allow only one blood cell at a time to pass through them. Don't confuse aort/o, meaning aorta, atri/o, meaning atrium, arteri/o, meaning artery, and arteriol/o, meaning arteriole.

Your heart is about the size of your fist. It is located in the mediastinum of the thoracic cavity, slightly to the left of the midline. The pointed tip (apex) rests just above the diaphragm. The area of the chest wall anterior to the heart is called the precordium (pre- = before + cordi/o = heart + -um = structure). The arteries of the heart (important in that they are the blood supply for the heart muscle) are called the coronary arteries. The two main coronary arteries are called the left and right coronary arteries. They supply a constant, uninterrupted blood flow to the heart. The areas of the heart wall that they feed are designated as inferior, lateral, anterior, and posterior.

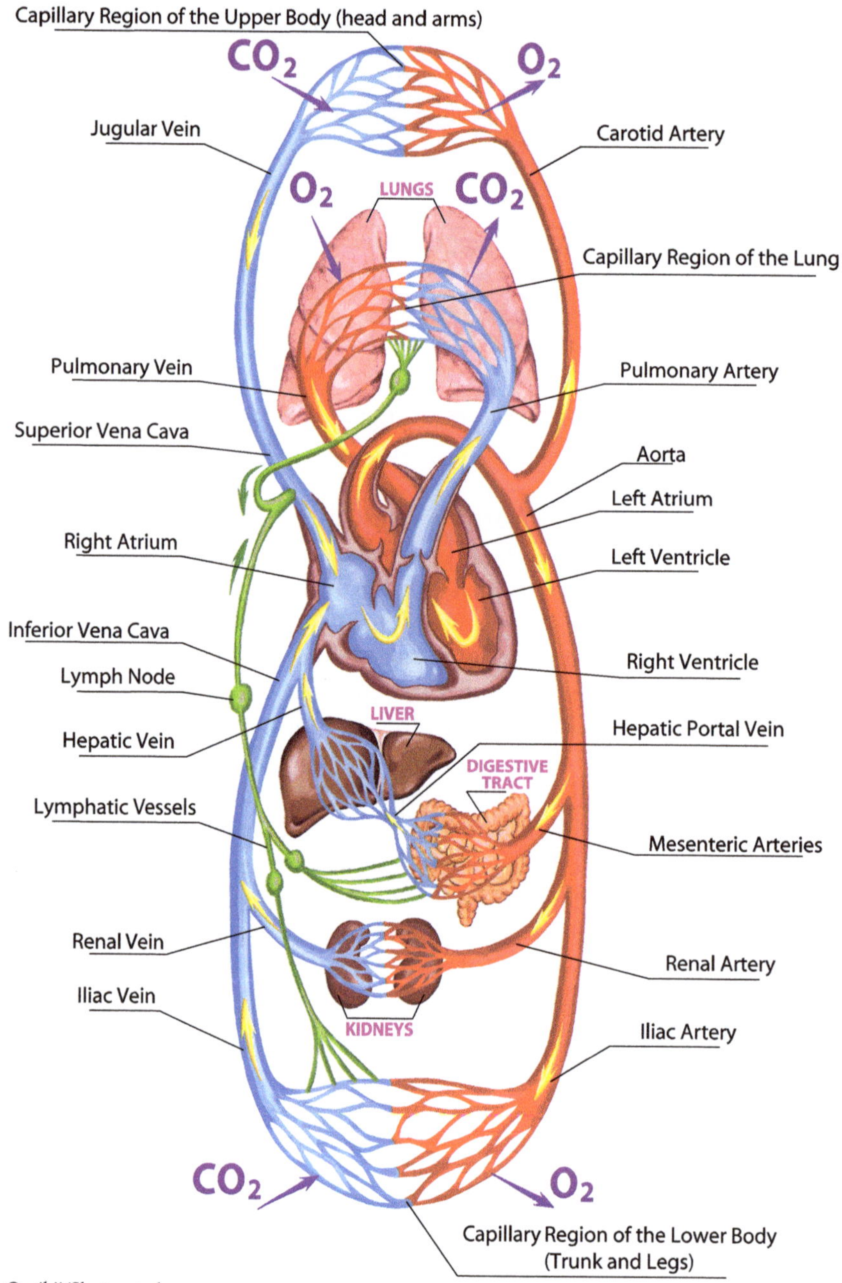

The heart has four chambers. The upper chambers are the atria (s. atrium) and the lower chambers are the ventricles. Both are divided into right-sided and left-sided chambers. Between the atria and ventricles and between the ventricles and vessels are valves that allow blood to flow in only one direction. The walls between the chambers are called the septa (s. septum). Between the atria, it is the interatrial (inter- = between + atri/o = atrium + -al = pertaining to) septum; and between the ventricles, it is the interventricular septum. Aside from the four chambers, the heart is composed of three layers. The endocardium (endo- = within + cardi/o = heart + -um = structure) is the thin

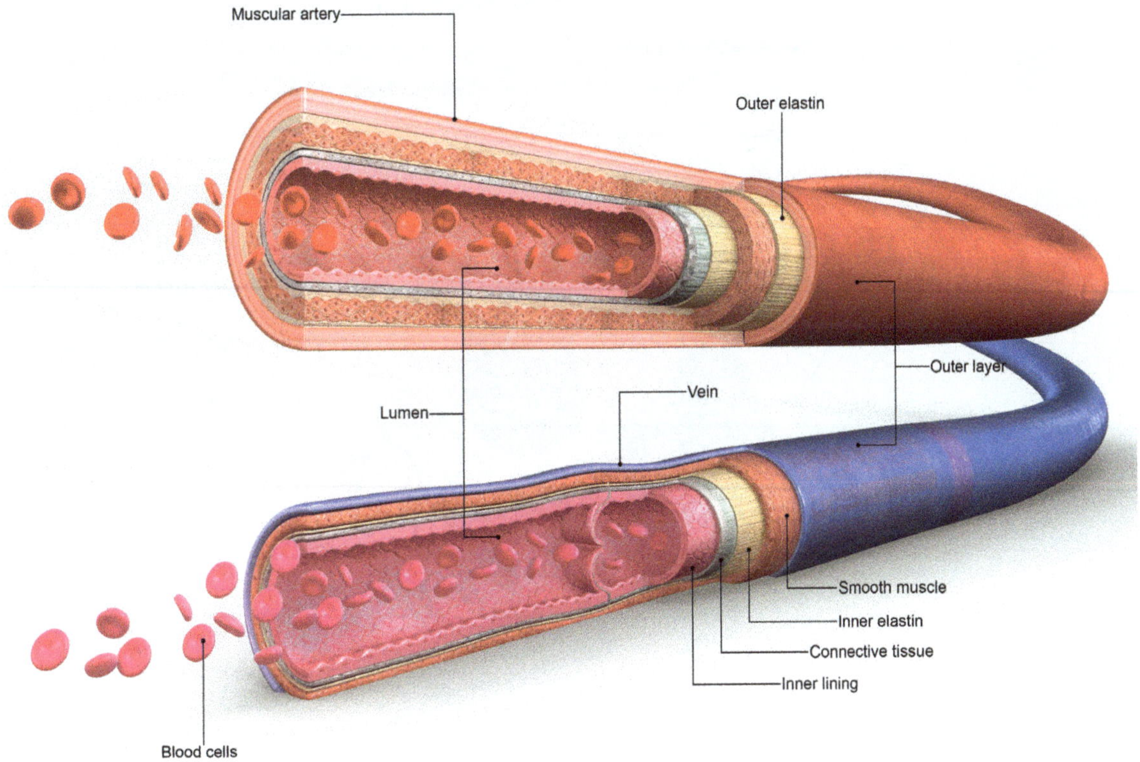

tissue that acts as a lining for each of the chambers. The myocardium (my/o = muscle + cardi/o = heart + -um = structure) is the cardiac muscle surrounding each of these chambers. The pericardium (peri- = surrounding + cardi/o = heart + -um = structure) is the double-folded layer of connective tissue that surrounds the heart. Its inner surface is called the visceral pericardium (viscer/o = organ, so it is the side that is closest to the organ of the heart), while the outer membrane, closest to the body wall, is called the parietal pericardium. Another name for the visceral pericardium is the epicardium (epi-=above, on top of), because is it the structure "on top of " the heart. The combining forms for these layers will be given as compound combining forms (endocardi/o, myocardi/o, and pericardi/o) now that you understand their derivation.

Trace the route of deoxygenated blood from the right atrium to the capillaries of the lungs.
Deoxygenated blood is returned to the heart through the superior and inferior venae cavae to the right atrium. When the right atrium contracts, the blood passes through the tricuspid valve into the right ventricle.

When the right ventricle contracts, the blood is pushed out into the pulmonary arteries to the lungs (note that these are the only arteries that carry deoxygenated blood).
These arteries deliver the deoxygenated blood to the capillaries of the lungs, where carbon dioxide leaves the blood and oxygen is picked up to begin the cycle of delivering oxygen to the cells over again.

The amount of blood expelled from the left ventricle compared with the total volume of blood filling the ventricle is referred to as the stroke volume and is a measure of the ejection

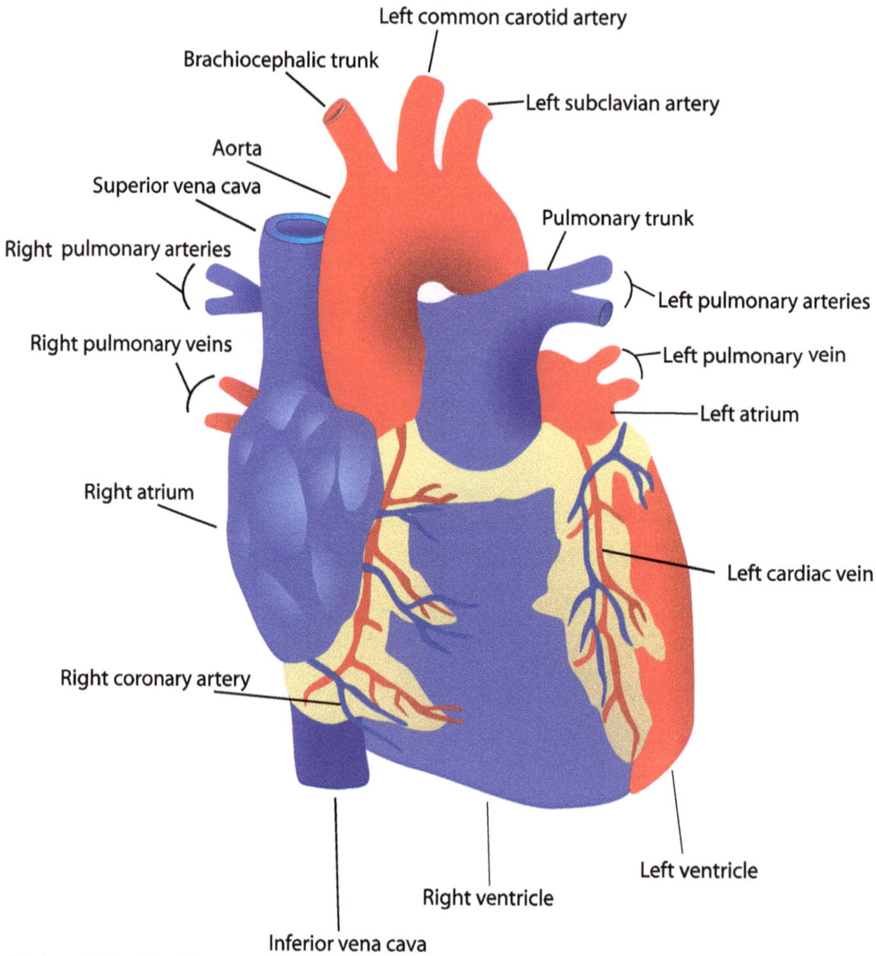

fraction of cardiac output. Think of these as a measure of the strength and efficiency of the heart muscle. The normal reading is around 65% for the ejection fraction; any percentage under that may indicate disease. The measure of the heart rate is calculated in beats per minute. Normal range is from 60 to 100 beats per minute.

The areas of measurement around the body are the pulse points. Take a look at the diagram to recognize these locations.

The cardiovascular system is dependent on the coordinated contractions and relaxations of the heart muscle. When this force, the blood pressure, is measured by an instrument termed a sphygmomanometer (a blood pressure cuff), the reading is measured as systole (the contractive phase) over diastole (the relaxation phase). Normal blood pressure is a range from 120 to 139/80 to 84. The timing of the contractions and relaxations is accomplished through the electrical pathways in the heart. The heartbeat begins at the sinoatrial node, the natural pacemaker of the heart. This initial signal causes the atria to contract.

The signal is then sent to the atrioventricular node, located at the base of the right atrium proximal to the interatrial (inter- = between) septum. From the atrioventricular node, the signal travels to the bundle of His (also called the atrioventricular bundle) in the interatrial septum. Its right and left bundle branches transmit the impulse of the Purkinje fibers in the right and left ventricles. Once the Purkinje fibers receive stimulation, they cause the ventricles to contract and force the blood out to the pulmonary arteries and the aorta.

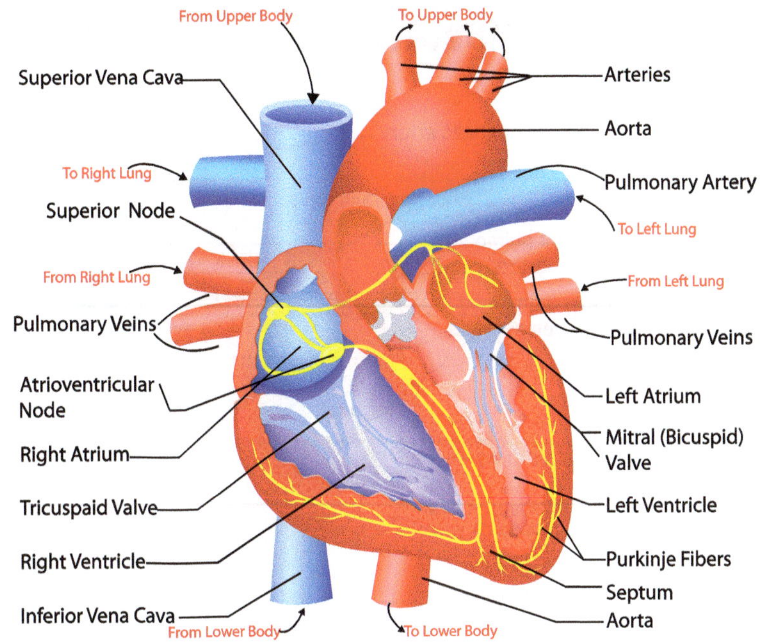

Normal electrical activity is referred to as normal sinus rhythm (NSR). An abnormality of the signals may result in an arrhythmia (an abnormal heartbeat).

Bradycardia (brady- = slow + -cardia = heart condition) is a slow heartbeat, with ventricular contractions less than 60 beats per minute. Tachycardia (tachy- = rapid + -cardia = heart condition) is a rapid heartbeat of more than 100 beats per minute. Cardiodynia (cardi/o = heart + -dynia = pain) is heart pain that may be described as atypical or ischemic. Atypical (a-= not) is a stabbing or burning pain that is variable in location and intensity and unrelated to exertion. Ischemic pain is a pressing, squeezing, or weight-like cardiac pain caused by decreased blood supply that usually lasts only minutes. Precordial (pre- = before, in front of + cordi/o = heart + -al = pertaining to) pain is pain in the area over the heart. Cardialgia and cardiodynia are synonyms.

Cardiomegaly (cardi/o = heart + -megaly = enlargement) is an enlargement of the heart.

Cyanosis (cyan/o = blue + -osis = abnormal condition) is a lack of oxygen in the blood, seen as a bluish or grayish discoloration of the skin, nail beds, and/or lips. Diaphoresis is the profuse secretion of sweat.

Claudication is cramp-like pains in the calves caused by poor circulation in the leg muscles.

Dyspnea (dys- difficult + -pnea = breathing); dyspnea on exertion (DOE) is difficult and/or painful breathing; if DOE, it is experienced when effort is expended.

Edema is an abnormal accumulation of fluid in the interstitial spaces of tissues.

Nausea is a sensation that accompanies the urge to vomit, but does not always lead to vomiting. Emesis is the forcible or involuntary emptying of the stomach through the mouth. A bruit is an abnormal sound heard when an artery is auscultated. It is usually a blowing or swishing sound, higher pitched than a murmur. A murmur is an abnormal heart sound heard during systole, diastole, or both, which may be described as a gentle blowing, fluttering, or humming sound. Pallor is a paleness of the skin and/or mucous membranes. On darker pigmented skin, it may be noted on the inner surfaces of the lower eyelids or the nail beds. Ischemia is a lack of blood in a body part due to blockage or constriction that interferes with normal blood flow.

Palpitations are the pounding or racing of the heart, such that the patient is aware of his or her heartbeat. Pulmonary congestion (pulmon/o = lung + -ary = pertaining to) is an excessive amount of blood in the pulmonary vessels. It is usually associated with the heart failure. Shortness of breath

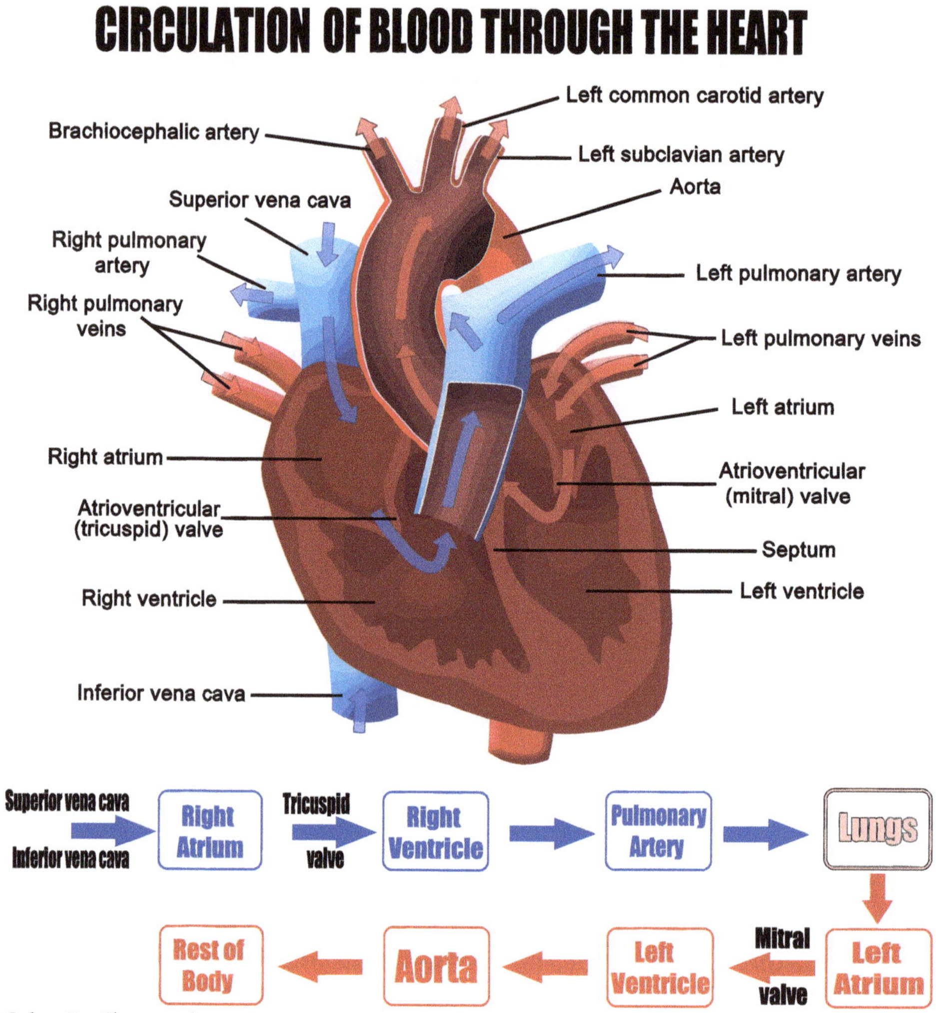

(SOB) is breathless; air hunger. Syncope is fainting, a loss of consciousness. A thrill is a fine vibration felt by the examiner on palpation. Venous distension is enlarged or swollen veins. Be careful! Do not confuse palpation, which means examination by touch, and palpitation, which means a pounding or racing of the heart.

Coarctation of the aorta is a congenital cardiac anomaly characterized by a localized narrowing of the aorta. Coarctation is another term for a narrowing.

Patent ductus arteriosus (PDA) is an abnormal opening between the pulmonary artery and the aorta caused by failure of the fetal ductus arteriosus to close after birth, most often in premature infants. Patent means open. Occluded means closed (or blocked).

A septal defect (sept/o = septum, wall + -al = pertaining to) is any congenital abnormality of the walls between the heart chambers. An atrial septal defect (ASD) is a hole in the wall between the upper chambers of the heart. A ventricular septal defect (VSD) is a hole in the wall between the lower two chambers of the heart.

Tetralogy of Fallot (tetra- = four + -logy = study of) is a congenital cardiac anomaly that consists of four defects: pulmonic stenosis; ventricular septal defect; malposition of the aorta, so that

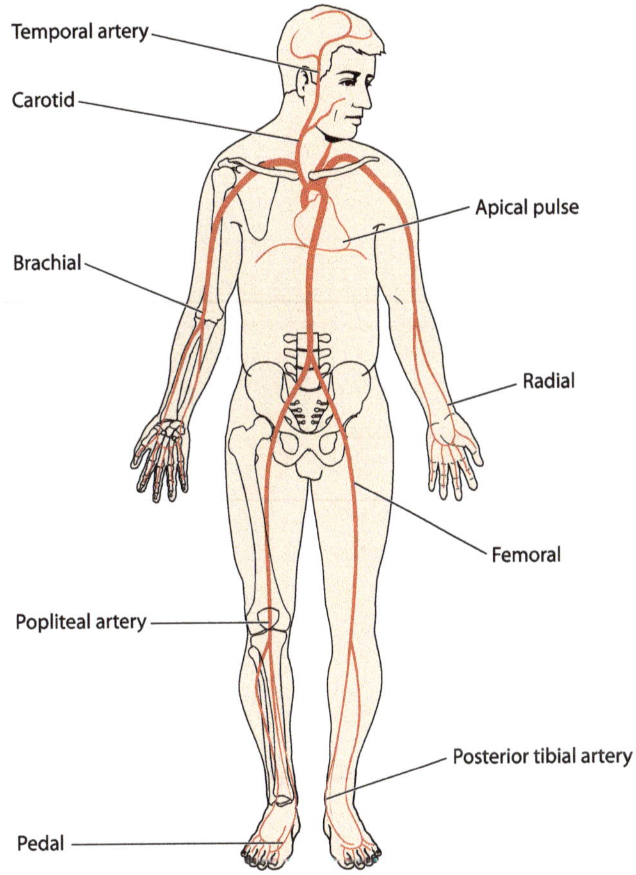

© Blamb/Shutterstock.com

it arises from the septal defect or the right ventricle; and right ventricular hypertrophy.

Aortic stenosis (stenosis = narrowing) is a narrowing of the aortic valve, which may be acquired or congenital. Mitral stenosis is a narrowing of the valve between the left atrium and left ventricle caused by adhesions on the leaflets of the valve, usually the result of recurrent episodes of rheumatic endocarditis. Left atrial hypertrophy develops and may be followed by right-sided heart failure and pulmonary edema (cor pulmonale). The term *mitral* is derived from the appearance of the valve and its similarity to a bishop's miter, or hat. Tricuspid stenosis is a relatively uncommon narrowing of the tricuspid valve associated with lesions of other valves caused by rheumatic fever. Symptoms include jugular vein distension and pulmonary congestion.

Mitral regurgitation is a backflow of blood from the left ventricle into the left atrium in systole across a diseased valve. It may be the result of congenital valve abnormalities, rheumatic fever, or mitral valve prolapse. Mitral valve prolapse (pro- forward + -lapse fall) is the protrusion of one or both cusps of the mitral valve back into the left atrium during ventricular systole. Orthopnea (orth/o = straight, upright + -pnea = breathing) is a condition in which a person must sit or stand to breathe comfortably. Valvulitis is an inflammatory condition of a valve, especially a cardiac valve, caused most commonly by rheumatic fever and less frequently by bacterial endocarditis or syphilis. Results are stenoses and obstructed blood flow.

Dysrhythmia (dys- abnormal + rhythm/o = rhythm + -ia = condition) is an abnormal heartbeat. An arrhythmia (a- without) is a synonym.

Ectopic beats (ec- out of + top/o = place + -ic = pertaining to) are heartbeats that occur outside of a normal rhythm.

- Atrial ectopic beats are irregular contractions of the atria. These are also termed *premature atrial contractions* (PAC).
- Ventricular ectopic beats are irregular contractions of the ventricles. These are also called *premature ventricular contractions* (PVC). These are not always considered pathologic.

Fibrillation is an extremely rapid and irregular contraction (300–600/min) that occurs with or without an underlying cardiovascular disorder, such as coronary artery disease.

- Atrial fibrillation is the most common type of cardiac arrhythmia. It is associated with excessive alcohol consumption.
- Ventricular fibrillation is rapid, irregular contractions that may be fatal unless reversed.

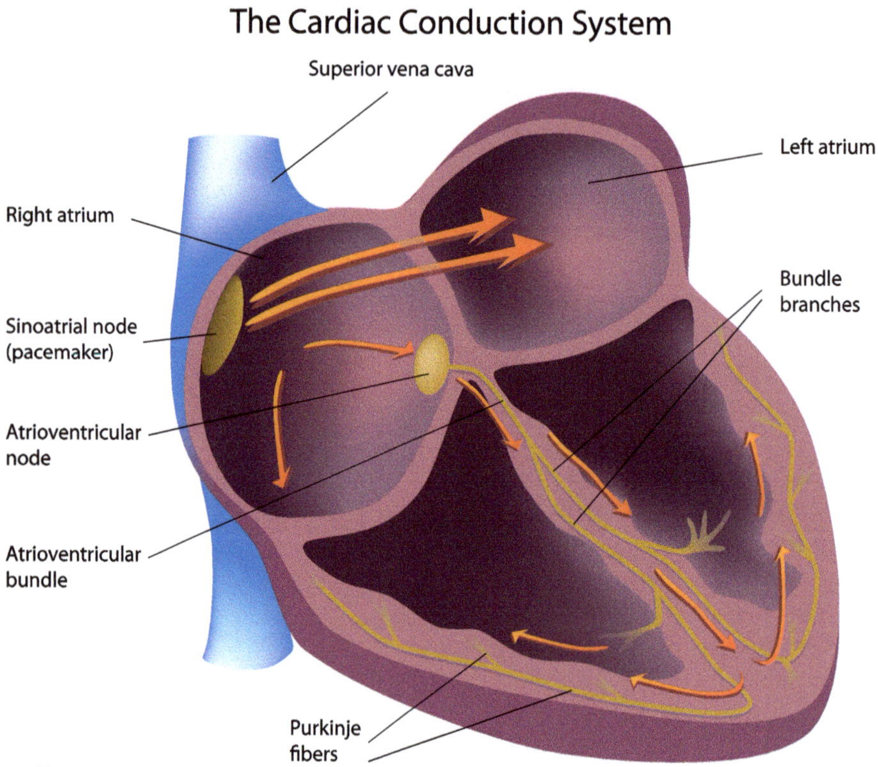

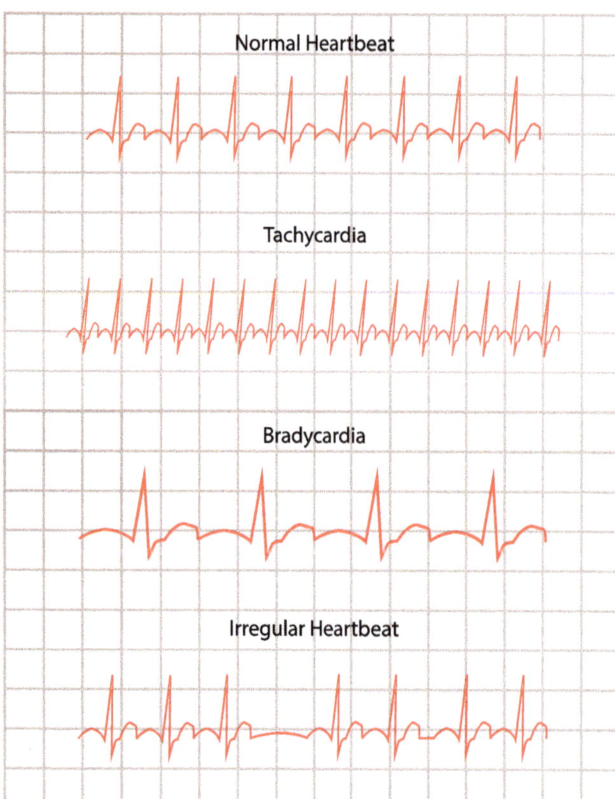

Flutter is extremely rapid but regular heartbeats (250–350/min). Atrial flutter is an extremely rapid, but regular atrial rhythm. Heart block is the result of a lack of electrical communication between the atria and the ventricles. It is also called atrioventricular block. Bundle branch block is an incomplete electrical conduction in the bundle branches, either on the left or on the right. Sick sinus syndrome is any abnormality of the sinus node; it may necessitate the placement of an implantable pacemaker. Ventricular tachycardia (tachy- rapid + -cardia = heart condition) is a condition of ventricular contractions that are greater than 100 beats per minute.

Angina pectoris (pector/o = chest + -is = structure) is paroxysmal chest pain that is often accompanied by shortness of breath and a sensation of impending doom.

Coronary artery disease (CAD) (coron/o = heart, crown) is an accumulation and hardening of plaque in the coronary arteries that eventually can deprive the heart

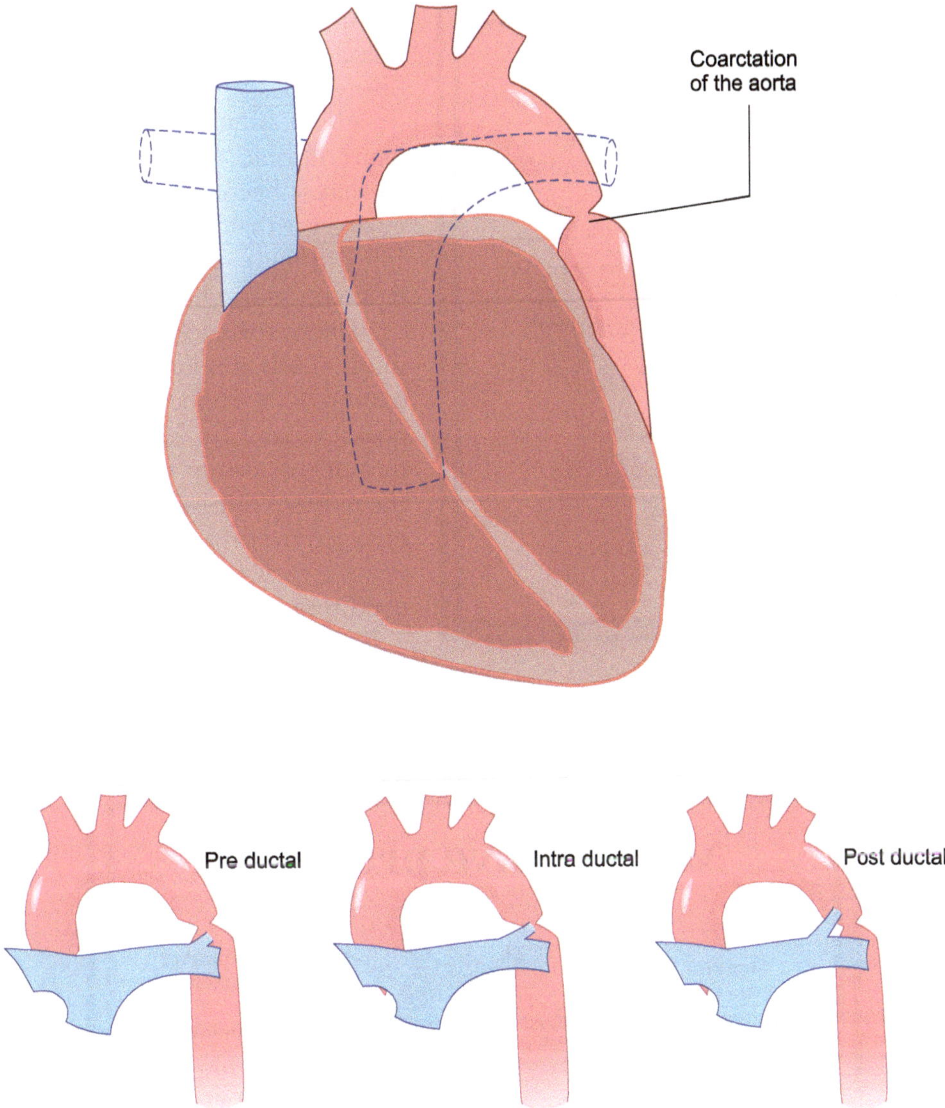

© ellepigrafica/Shutterstock.com

muscle of oxygen, leading to angina. CAD is the leading cause of death in both sexes in the United States, accounting for one-third of all deaths each year. Myocardial infarction (MI) is cardiac tissue death that occurs when the coronary arteries are occluded (blocked) by an atheroma, a mass of fat or lipids on the wall of an artery, or a blood clot caused by an atheroma, and thus are unable to carry enough oxygenated blood to the heart muscle. Depending on the area affected, the patient may die if enough heart muscle is destroyed. This is commonly called a heart attack. A silent heart attack is one that the patient is not aware of, usually because it destroys such a small amount of tissue. A massive heart attack is one that destroys a large amount of tissue, often enough to be fatal.

Be careful! Infarction refers to tissue death. An infraction refers to a breaking, as in an incomplete bone fracture.

Cardiac tamponade is a compression of the heart caused by fluid in the pericardial sac.

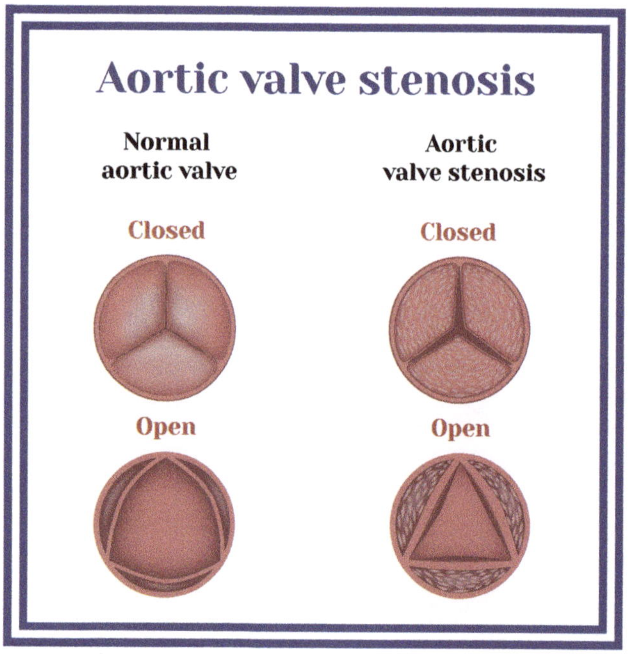

Cardiomyopathy (cardiomy/o = heart muscle + -pathy = diseases) is a progressive disorder of the ventricles of the heart.

Heart failure (HF) is an inability of the heart muscle to pump blood efficiently, so that it becomes overloaded. The heart enlarges with unpumped blood and the lungs fill with fluid. This was previously referred to as congestive heart failure (CHF).

Endocarditis (endocardi/o = endocardium + -itis = inflammation) is an inflammation of the endocardium and heart valves, characterized by lesions and caused by a number of different microbes. Although the number of cases of endocarditis has not changed over the past few decades, twice as many men as women are diagnosed with this condition.

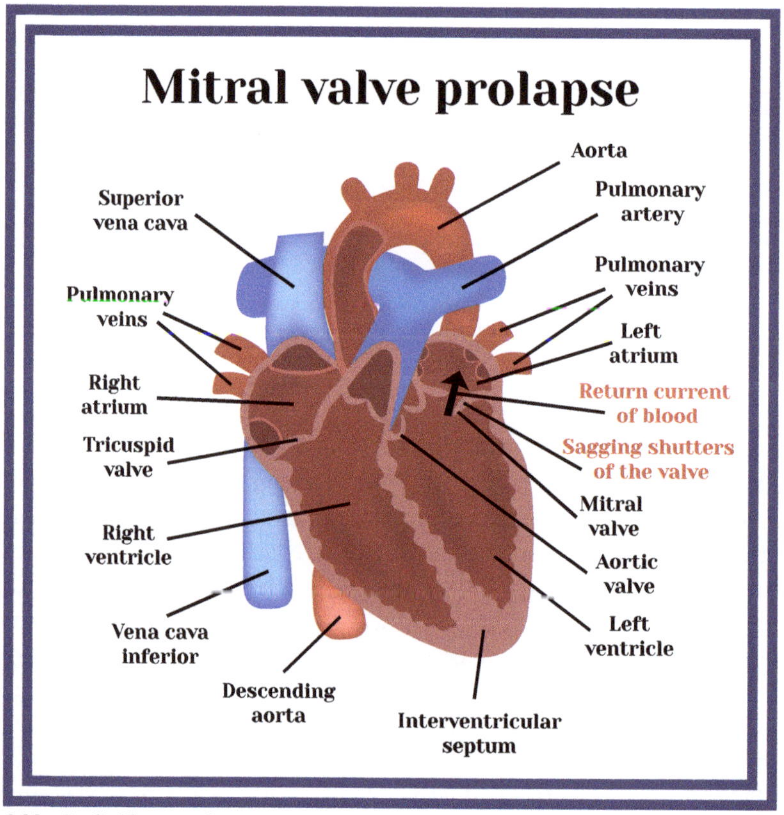

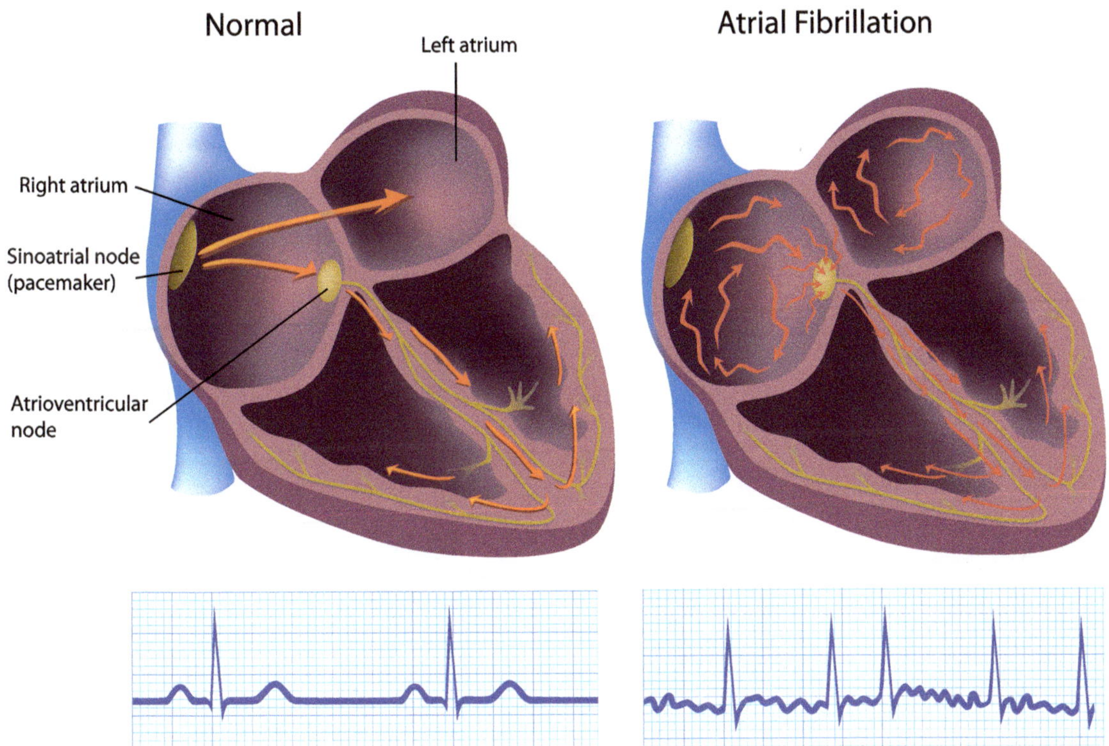

© Alila Medical Media/Shutterstock.com

Pericarditis (pericardi/o = pericardium + -itis = inflammation) is an inflammation of the sac surrounding the heart, with the possibility of pericardial effusion.

Arteriosclerosis (arteri/o = artery + -sclerosis = abnormal condition of hardening) is a disease in which the arterial walls become thickened and lose their elasticity, without the presence of atheromas (ather/o = fat, plaque + -oma = mass). Arteriosclerosis is the leading cause of morbidity and mortality in the United States today.

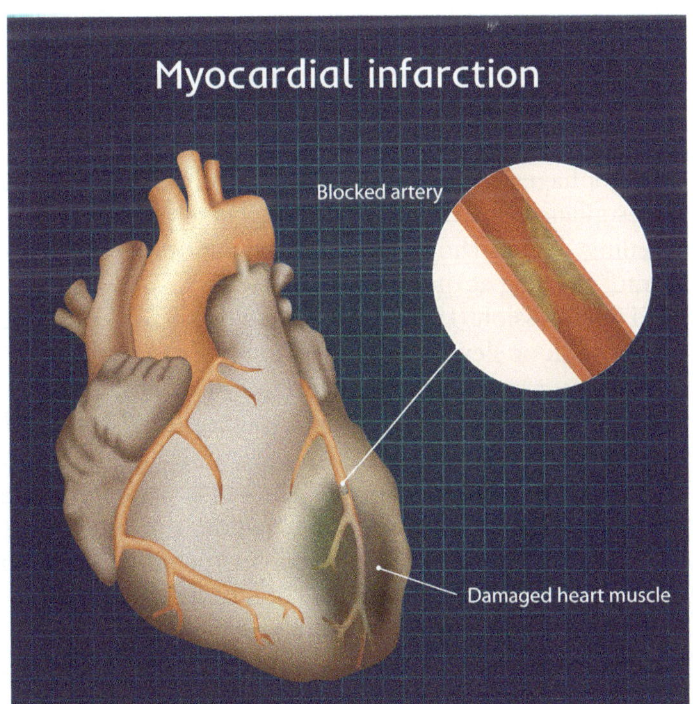

© Veronika Zakharova/Shutterstock.com

Atherosclerosis (ather/o = fat, plaque + -sclerosis = abnormal condition of hardening) is a form of arteriosclerosis in which medium and large arteries have atheromas, which can reduce or obstruct blood flow. Patients with peripheral atherosclerosis

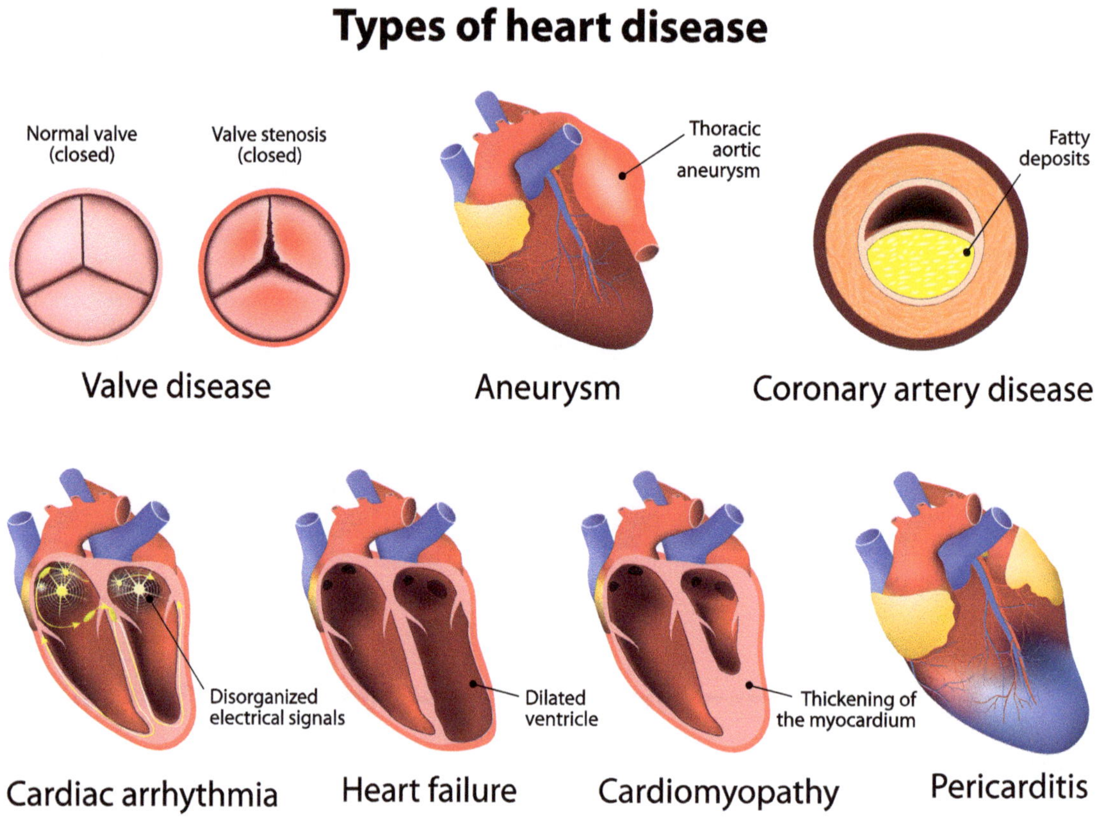

complain of intermittent claudication. An aneurysm is a localized dilation of an artery caused by a congenital or acquired weakness in the wall of the vessel. The acquired causes may be arteriosclerosis, trauma, infection, and/or inflammation.

Esophageal varices (varic/o = dilated vein) are varicose veins that appear at the lower end of the esophagus as a result of portal hypertension; they are superficial and may cause ulceration and bleeding. Hemorrhoids are varicose conditions of the external or internal rectal veins that cause painful swelling at the anus.

Hypertension (HTN) (hyper- excessive + tens/o = stretching + -ion = process of) is a condition of high or elevated blood pressure, also known as arterial hypertension. It occurs in two main forms: primary (or essential) hypertension, which has no identifiable cause; and secondary hypertension, which occurs in response to another disorder. Malignant hypertension is very high blood pressure that results in organ damage. Almost one in five Americans has been diagnosed with HTN. Hypotension (hypo- below, deficient + tens/o = stretching + -ion = process of) is a condition of below normal blood pressure. Orthostatic hypotension occurs when a patient experiences an episode of low blood pressure upon rising to a standing position. Peripheral arterial occlusion (occlus/o = blockage + ion = process of) is the blockage of blood flow to the extremities. Acute or chronic conditions may be present, but patients with both types of conditions are likely to have underlying atherosclerosis. Peripheral vascular disease (PVD) is any vascular disorder limited to the extremities. It may affect not only the arteries and veins but also the lymphatics.

Process of Arteriosclerosis

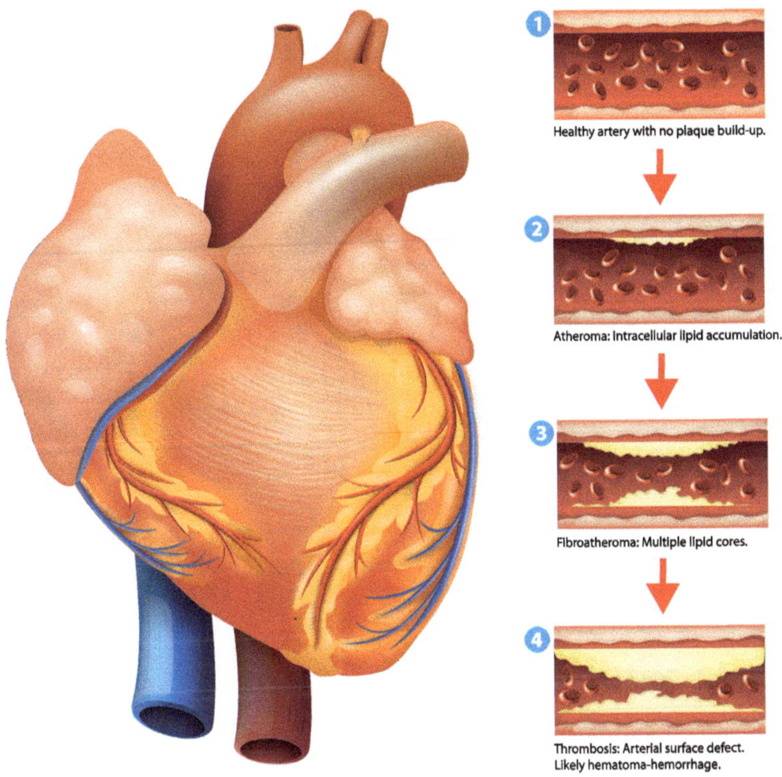

Thrombophlebitis (thromb/o = clotting, clot + phleb/o + vein + -itis = inflammation) is inflammation of either deep veins (deep vein thrombosis, or DVT) or superficial veins (superficial vein thrombosis, or SVT), with the formation of one or more blood clots.

Varicose veins are elongated, dilated superficial veins (varices) with incompetent valves that permit reverse blood flow. These veins may appear in various parts of the anatomy, but the term varicose vein(s) has been reserved for those in the lower extremities.

Vasculitis (vascul/o = vessel + -itis = inflammation) is an inflammation of the blood vessels. It is also called angiitis.

Blood pressure is a measure of systolic pressure over diastolic pressure. The instrument used for this measure is a sphygmomanometer [literally, an instrument to measure (-meter) pulse (sphygm/o) pressure (man/o)].

Auscultation (listening) and percussion (tapping) is a diagnostic technique used to detect differences in density within a body cavity. The instrument that amplifies the sounds within the body is a stethoscope (steth/o = chest + -scope = instrument to view, although here it is to examine).

Echocardiography (echo- = reverberation + cardi/o = heart + -graphy = process of recording) is the use of ultrasonic waves directed through the heart to study the structure and motion of the heart. Transesophageal echocardiography (trans- = through) images the heart through a transducer introduced into the esophagus. Exercise stress tests are images of the heart during exercise on a treadmill, with the use of radioactive thallium.

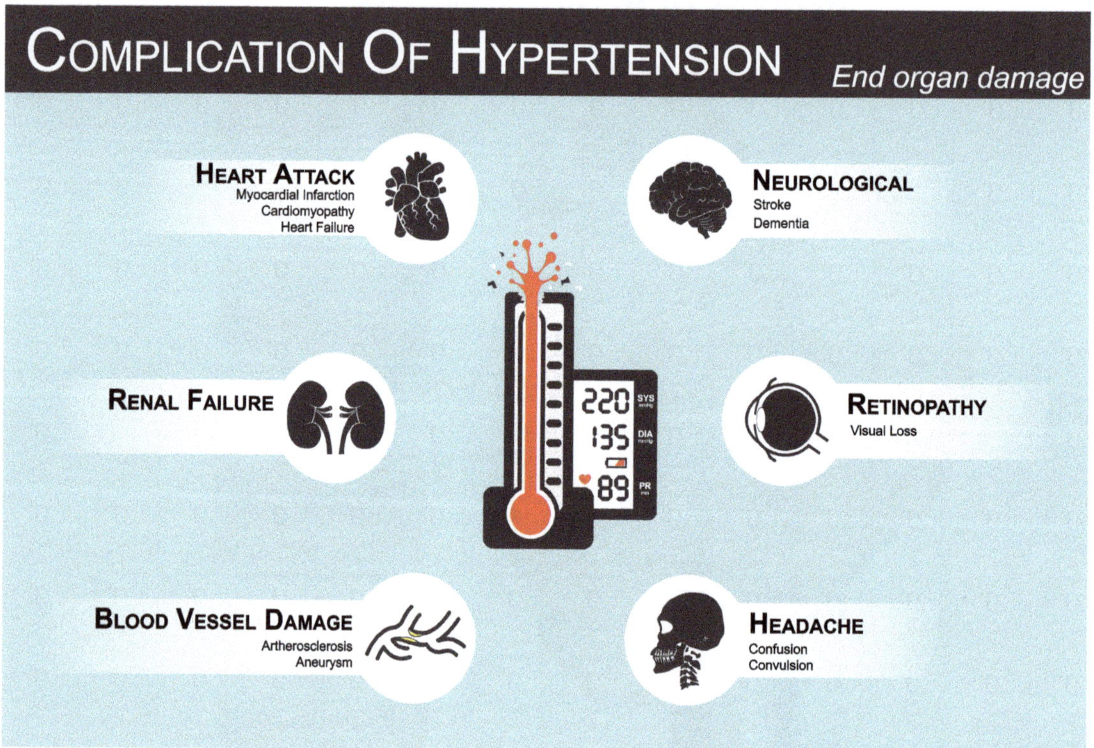

© Puwadol Jaturawutthichai/Shutterstock.com

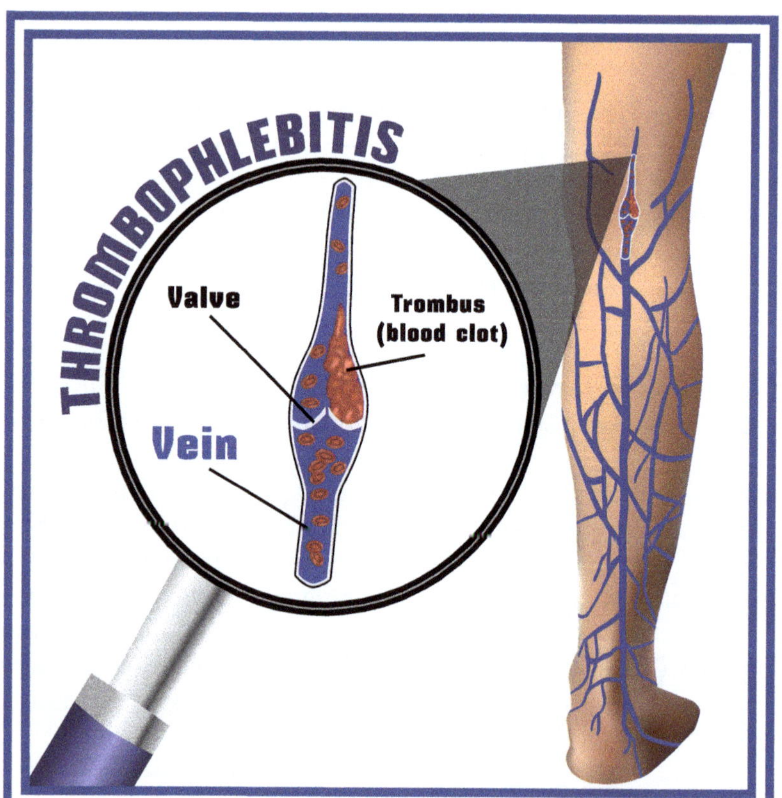

© Mrs_Bazilio/Shutterstock.com

Magnetic resonance imaging is a computerized imaging that uses radiofrequency pulses in a magnetic field to detect areas of myocardial infarction (tissue death), stenoses (areas of narrowing), and areas of blood flow.

Multiple-gated acquisition (MUGA) scans are noninvasive methods of imaging a beating heart by tagging RBCs with a radioactive substance. A gamma camera captures the outline of the chambers of the heart as the blood passes through them.

Myocardial perfusion imaging is the use of radionuclides to diagnose CAD, valvular or congenital heart disease, and cardiomyopathy. Positron emission tomography is a computerized nuclear medicine procedure that uses inhaled or injected radioactive substances to help identify how much a patient will benefit from revascularization procedures. Radiography, in the form of chest x-rays, is used to evaluate the size and shape of the heart in posteroanterior and lateral views. Phlebography (phleb/o = vein + -graphy = process of recording) is an x-ray of a vein after the introduction of a contrast dye.

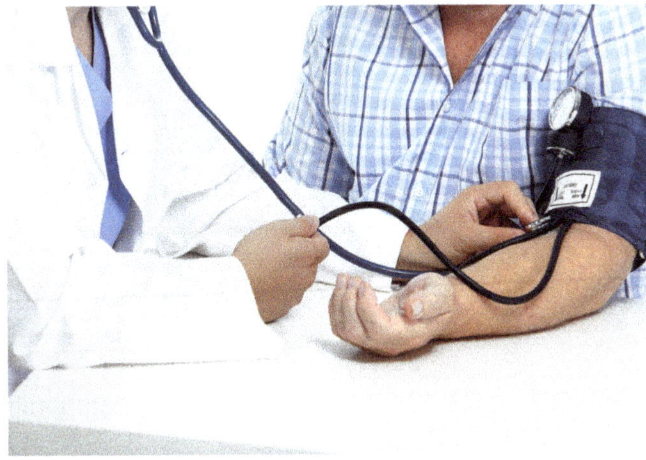

© kurhan/Shutterstock.com

Cardiac catheterization is the threading of a catheter (thin tube) into the heart to collect diagnostic information about structures in the heart, coronary arteries, and great vessels; it is also used to aid in the treatment of CAD, congenital abnormalities, and heart failure.

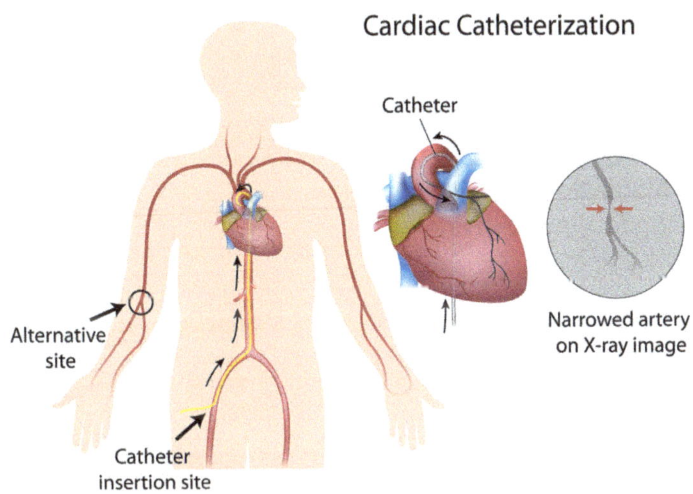

© Alila Medical Media/Shutterstock.com

A Swan-Ganz catheter is a long, thin cardiac catheter with a tiny balloon at the tip that is fed into the femoral artery near the groin and extended up to the left ventricle. This instrument is used to determine left ventricular function by measuring pulmonary capillary wedge pressure. Fluoroscopy is an x-ray procedure that allows visualization of structures in real time directly on a monitor screen. The combining form fluor/o means to flow, as this imaging procedure is a "flow" of images, not a static image.

Electrocardiography (electr/o = electricity + cardi/o = heart + -graphy = process of recording) is a recording of electrical impulses of the heart as wave deflections of a needle on an instrument called an electrocardiograph (-graph = instrument to record). The record, or recording, is called an electrocardiogram. A Holter monitor is a portable electrocardiograph that is worn to record the reaction of the heart to daily activities.

Cardiac enzymes tests are blood tests that measure the amount of cardiac enzymes characteristically released during a myocardial infarction. They determine the amount of lactate dehydrogenase (LDH) and creatine phosphokinase (CK or CPK) in the blood.

A lipid profile is a blood test to measure the lipids (cholesterol and triglycerides) in the circulating blood. Phlebotomy (phleb/o = vein + -tomy = incision) is the opening of a vein to withdraw a blood sample. It is also referred to as venipuncture.

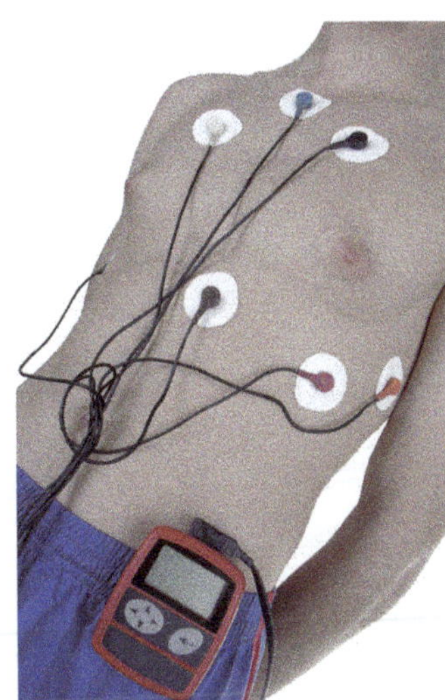

© papa1266/Shutterstock.com

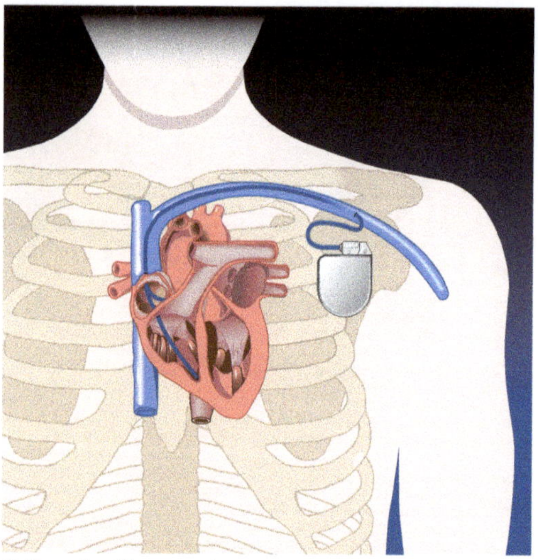

© Alexonline/Shutterstock.com

A carotid endarterectomy (end- = within + arter/o = artery + -ectomy = removal) is the removal of the atheromatous plaque lining the carotid artery to increase blood flow and leave a smooth surface. The procedure is done to prevent thrombotic occlusions (blockages).

A thromboendarterectomy is the removal of a blood clot along with part of the lining of the artery and possibly associated plaque.

Cardiac pacemakers are small, battery-operated devices that help the heart beat in a regular rhythm. They can be either internal (permanent) or external (temporary).

An automatic implantable cardioverter-defibrillator (AICD) is a device that is implanted in the chest to monitor the heartbeat and correct it if needed (speed it up or slow it down).

A cardiac defibrillator is either an external or an implantable device that provides an electronic shock to the heart to restore a normal rhythm.

Cardiopulmonary resuscitation (CPR) is a manual external cardiac massage and artificial respiration used to restart the heartbeat and breathing of a patient.

Coronary artery bypass graft (CABG) surgery is an open-heart procedure in which a piece of a blood vessel from another location is grafted onto one of the coronary arteries to reroute blood around a blockage.

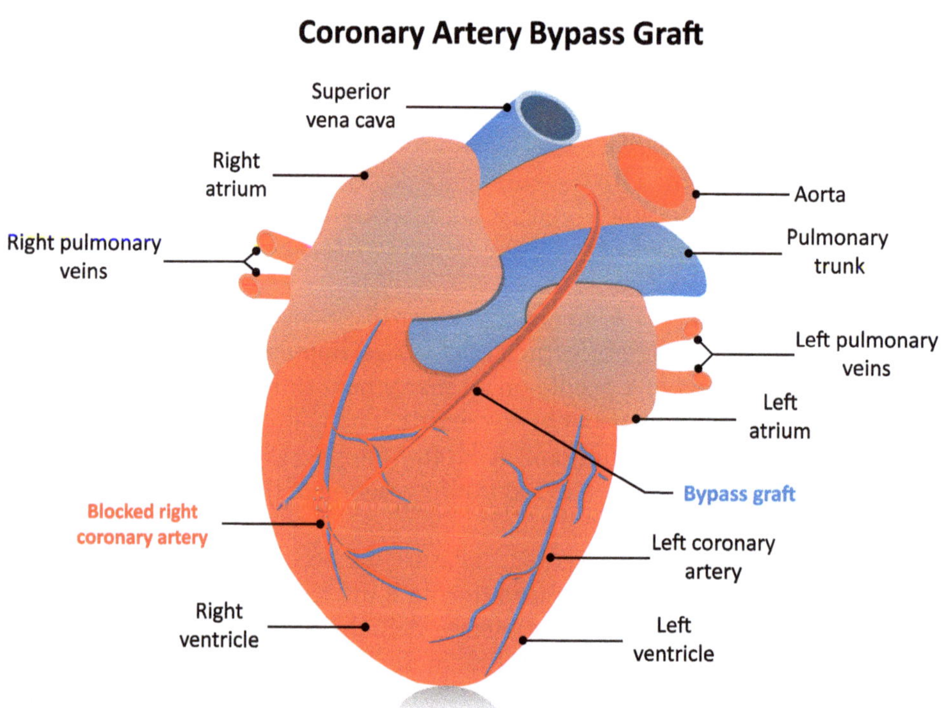

© joshya/Shutterstock.com

Heart transplantation is the removal of a diseased heart and transplantation of a donor heart when cardiac disease can no longer be treated by any other means.

A left ventricular assist device is a mechanical pump device that assists a patient's weakened heart by pulling blood from the left ventricle into the pump and then ejecting it out into the aorta. LVADs may be used on those patients awaiting a transplant.

A minimally invasive direct coronary artery bypass is a surgical procedure in which the heart is still beating while a minimal incision is made over the blocked coronary artery and an artery from the chest wall is used as the bypass.

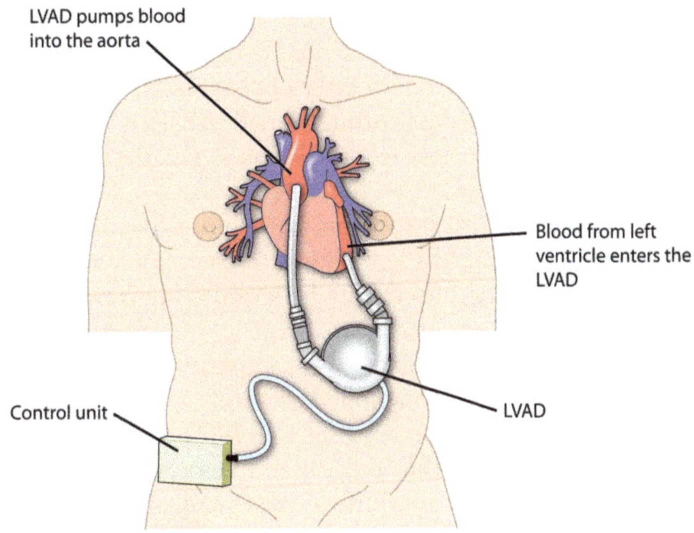

© Blamb/Shutterstock.com

Percutaneous (per- through + cutane/o = skin + -ous = pertaining to) transluminal (trans- = through + lumin/o = lumen + -al = pertaining to) coronary angioplasty (angi/o = vessel + -plasty = surgical repair) is a surgical procedure in which a catheter is threaded into the coronary artery that is affected by atherosclerotic heart disease. The balloon at the tip of the catheter is inflated and deflated to compress the plaque against the wall of the artery and increase blood flow. Stents (wire mesh tubes) are placed in the arteries and used to prop them open after the angioplasty.

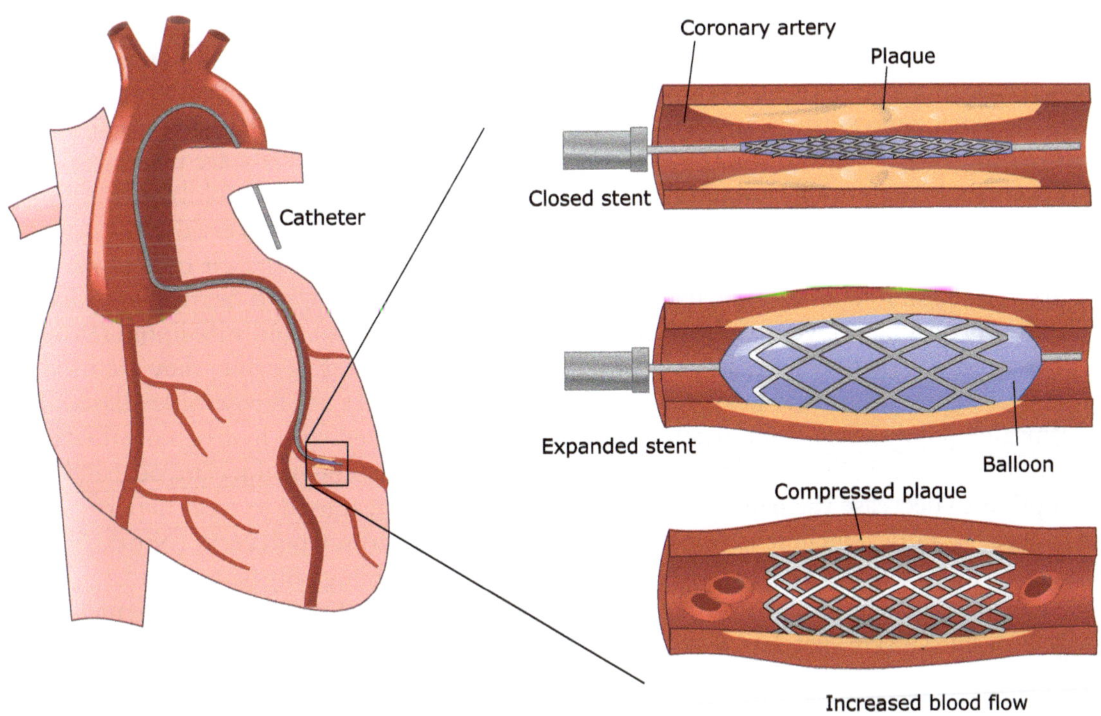

© ellepigrafica/Shutterstock.com

Pericardiocentesis (pericardi/o = pericardium + -centesis = surgical puncture) is an aspiration of fluid from the pericardium to treat cardiac tamponade.

A port-access coronary artery bypass is a procedure in which the heart is stopped and bypass surgery is accomplished through small incisions in the chest.

Radiofrequency catheter ablation is the destruction of abnormal cardiac electrical pathways causing arrhythmias.

Transmyocardial revascularization is a procedure used to relieve severe angina in a patient who cannot tolerate a CABG or PTCA. With a laser, a series of holes is made in the heart tissue in the hope of increasing blood flow by stimulating new blood vessels to grow. Angiogenesis (angi/o = vessel + -genesis = production).

Valvuloplasty (valvul/o = valve + -plasty = surgical repair) is the repair of a stenosed heart valve with the use of a balloon-tipped catheter.

Angiotensin (angi/o = vessel + tens/o = stretching + -in=substance) converting enzyme (ACE) inhibitors are drugs that relax blood vessels by preventing the formation of the vasoconstrictor angiotensin II. This inhibition causes a decrease in water retention and blood pressure and an improvement in cardiac output. ACE inhibitors are commonly used to treat hypertension and heart failure. Examples are Lisinopril (Prinivil), enalapril (Vasotec), and quinapril (Accupril).

Angiotensin II receptor blockers (ARBs) are drugs that lower blood pressure by inhibiting angiotensin II from binding its action sites. Examples include irbesartan (Avapro) and valsartan (Diovan).

Antiarrhythmic drugs work via various mechanisms to treat cardiac arrhythmias and restore normal sinus rhythm. Examples include digoxin (Lanoxin).

Anticoagulants (anti- = against + coagulant = clotting) are drugs used to prevent the formation of blood clots. Examples are warfarin (Coumadin) and heparin.

Antihyperlipidemics (anti- = against + hyper- = excessive + lipid/o = fat + -emic = pertaining to blood condition) are drugs that lower cholesterol levels to reduce the risk of heart attack or stroke. There are five different types: fibrates (Gemfibrozil), HMG-CoA reductase inhibitors or "statins" (Simvastatin), bile acid sequestrants (Cholestyramine), niacin, and ezetimibe. Beta-blockers are drugs that depress the heart rate and the force of heart contractions by decreasing the effectiveness of the nerve impulses to the cardiovascular system. They typically are prescribed to treat angina pectoris, hypertension, and cardiac arrhythmias. Examples are propranolol (Inderal), atenolol (Tenormin), and metoprolol (Lopressor). Calcium channel blockers (CCBs) are drugs that decrease myocardial oxygen demand by inhibiting the flow of calcium to smooth muscle cells of the heart to cause arterial relaxation. They are used to treat angina, hypertension, and heart failure. Examples are diltiazem (Cardizem), verapamil (Calan), amlodipine (Norvasc), and nifedipine (Procardia). Diuretics are drugs that promote the excretion of sodium and water as urine; they are used in the treatment of hypertension and heart failure. Examples of diuretics are furosemide (Lasix), hydrochlorothiazide (Hydrodiuril), and triamterene (Maxzide, combined with hydrochlorothiazide).

Nitrates (antianginals) are drugs that relax blood vessels and reduce myocardial oxygen consumption to decrease the pain of angina pectoris; they are also used to treat hypertension and heart failure. Examples include isosorbide dinitrate (Isordil) and nitroglycerin (Nitro, Nitro-dur, and Transderm-Nitro). Nitroglycerin (NTG) is administered sublingually (sub- = under + lingu/o = tongue), intravascularly (intra- = within + vascul/o = vessel), or through a transdermal (trans- = through + derm/o = skin) patch.

Discuss the different routes of administration for the delivery of antianginals.

Thrombolytics (thromb/o = clot + -lytic = pertaining to breaking down) are drugs that aid in the dissolution of blood clots. "Clot busters" are used to treat obstructing coronary thrombi (clots). Examples are tissue plasminogen activator (tPA), streptokinase, alteplase, reteplase, and tenecteplase.

The heart is one of the most complex organs besides the brain. The hearts ability to control blood flow, generate electricity, conduct electricity, and act on that electricity. Therefore over the course of a year, your heart beats between 31,536,000 and 42,048,000 times. Therefore we should protect our heart.

CHAPTER 8

Respiratory

The respiratory system is made up of the nose, pharynx, larynx, trachea, bronchi, and lungs. Its primary function is to supply oxygen for tissue cells to use and to take away their waste or carbon dioxide. To do this, the body goes through the act of respiration, which consists of internal and external processes. External respiration is the process by which the lungs are ventilated, and oxygen and carbon dioxide are exchanged between the air in the lungs and the blood within capillaries of the aveoli. Internal respiration is the process by which oxygen and carbon dioxide are exchanged between the blood in tissue capillaries and the cells in the body.

Oxygen is taken in and carbon dioxide is breathed out during respiration. On the route to the lungs, the air is filtered, warmed, and humidified. The respiratory system also assists in the regulation of the acidity/alkalinity of blood.

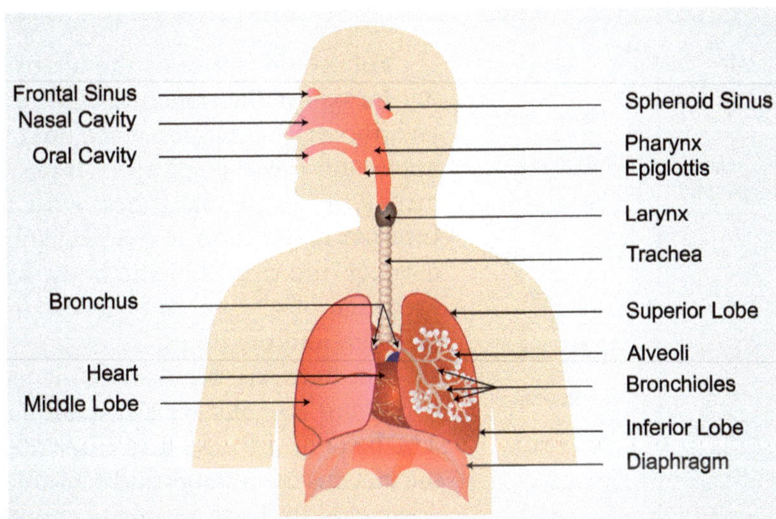

Functions of the Respiratory System

- □ Oxygen (ox/o, ox/i)
- □ Carbon dioxide (capn/o)
- □ Filtering, warming, humidifying air
- □ Regulation of blood pH
- □ Role in sound, speech, and olfaction

Inspiration (in- = in + spir/o = breathing), inhalation (hal/o = breathing). Expiration and exhalation (ex- = out). Note that the s of spir/o is dropped because of the x providing the sound of the s. The study of the lungs is pulmonology and the specialist is called a pulmonologist. The air enters the nose and travels down the pharynx, larynx, and trachea to the bronchi and the lungs. On inspiration, the diaphragm contracts, pulling air into the lungs. On expiration, the diaphragm relaxes, and air is expelled from the lungs.

- Upper respiratory tract
  - Nose (nas/o, rhin/o)
  - Pharynx (pharyng/o)
  - Larynx (laryng/o)
- Lower respiratory tract
  - Trachea (trache/o)
  - Bronchial tree (bronch/o, bronchi/o)
  - Lungs (pulmon/o, pneum/o, pneumon/o)
- Internal respiration vs. external respiration

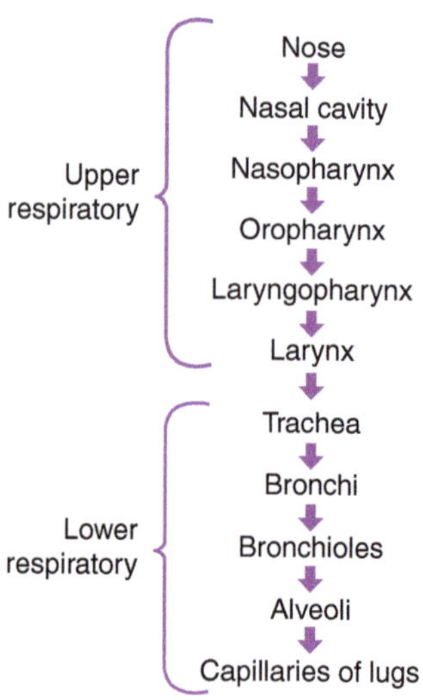

Follow the route of the air to the lungs and note the combining forms for the structures. Note the common names of the pharynx (throat) and larynx (voice box). Note the separation between the upper and lower respiratory tracts. Don't confuse bronchi/o, which means the bronchial tubes, with brachi/o, which means the arm. Internal respiration is the exchange of oxygen and carbon dioxide between the tissues of the body, whereas external respiration is the exchange of oxygen and carbon dioxide between the external environment and the lungs.

The nares are the nostrils, the nasal septum is the wall between the nares, and the cilia are the small hairs that line the respiratory tract. The hairs in the nose help filter the air as it enters the nose, whereas the mucous membranes and cilia are a means of keeping the tract clean, warm, and moist as air moves through the nasal cavity. The olfactory receptors are located in the nasal cavity.

The paranasal (para- = near) sinuses are the cavities in bone that are near the nose. Each of the four sinuses acquires its name from the bones in which it is located: the frontal, maxillary, sphenoid, and ethmoid.

The throat is divided into three sections:

The nasopharynx is directly behind the nose. The eustachian tube, which connects the ears to the throat, opens here. This is also the site of the pharyngeal tonsils (the adenoids), which consists of lymphatic tissue that helps prevent pathogens from entering through this opening. Be careful! The combining form salping/o means both eustachian tubes and fallopian tubes.

The oropharynx is the part of the throat that is directly behind the oral cavity (or/o = mouth). The palatine tonsils are the lymphatic tissues that guard this opening.

The laryngopharynx (also called the hypopharynx) is the part of the throat that is below the oropharynx and is close to the voice box, the larynx.

The larynx is the location of the vocal cords, which vibrate to produce speech as air passes back out through an opening in the larynx.

The epiglottis is a flap of cartilage at the opening to the larynx that closes access to the trachea (the windpipe) during swallowing so that food is routed to the esophagus and is kept from entering the trachea.

The lower respiratory system begins with the windpipe, which extends through the mediastinum (the space between the lungs). The trachea bifurcates (divides into two branches) at the carina and becomes the right and left bronchi. The bronchi divide into even smaller branches called bronchioles, which end in microscopic ducts capped by air sacs called alveoli (s. alveolus).

HUMAN DIGESTIVE SYSTEM

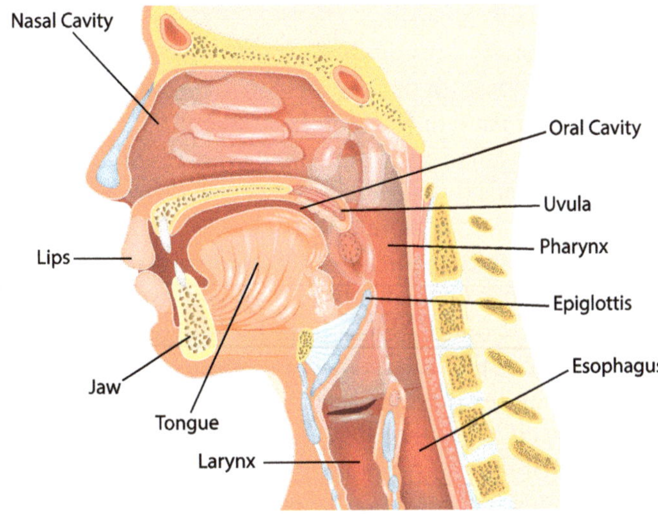

© Teguh Mujiono/Shutterstock.com

Each alveolus is in contact with a blood capillary to provide a means of exchange of oxygen and carbon dioxide. Each alveolus is coated with a substance called a surfactant that keeps the sac from collapsing.

The lungs are composed of sections called lobes. The right lung has three lobes whereas the left lung has only two.

The lungs are enclosed in a double-folded, serous membrane called a pleura. The side of the membrane that coats the lungs is the visceral pleura (viscer/o = organ), whereas the parietal pleura is the side that is closer to the body wall. The two sides of the pleural membrane enclose a small amount of fluid that serves to reduce friction and facilitate the contraction and expansion of the lungs.

The muscles that are responsible for respiration are the diaphragm, a large flat muscle that is located between the thoracic and abdominal cavities, and the intercostal muscles (inter-= between + cost/o = rib), which are the muscles between the lungs.

Aphonia (a-=without + phon/o = sound) is a loss of the ability to produce sounds. Dysphonia (dys- = difficult), a term used to discuss a condition of hoarseness, is difficulty making sound. Cheyne-Stokes respiration is deep, rapid breathing followed by a period of apnea (a temporary lack of breathing). Clubbing is the abnormal enlargement of the distal (the far ends) phalanges as a result of diminished oxygen in the blood. Cyanosis (cyan/o = blue) is a discoloration of the skin and mucous membranes due to insufficient oxygenation of the blood. The color of the skin, nail beds, and/or mucous membranes may be blue (as the term describes) or gray, slate, or dark purple. Note that the "blueness" may appear as a gray shade in different

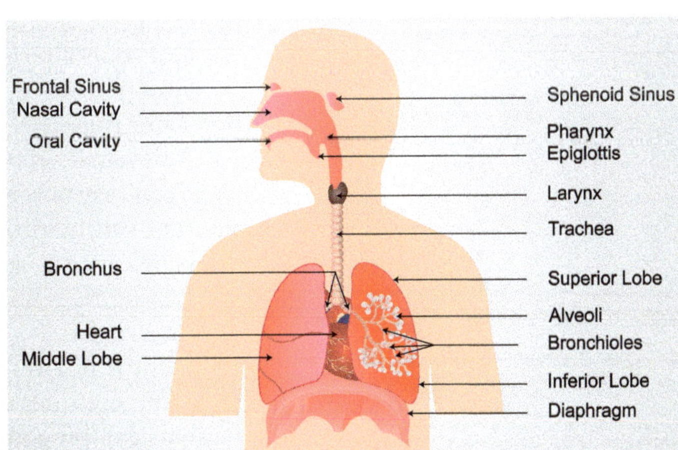

© stockshoppe/Shutterstock.com

shades of skin. Also note that it can be seen in the nailbeds and gingivae. Epistaxis is the medical term for a nosebleed.

Hemoptysis (-ptysis = spitting) is the coughing up of blood or blood-stained sputum.

Hypercapnia (hyper- = excessive + capn/o = carbon dioxide) is a condition of an excessive amount of carbon dioxide in the blood.

Hyperventilation is abnormally increased breathing.

Hypoxemia (hypo- = deficient + ox/o = oxygen + -emia = blood condition) is a condition of deficient oxygen in the blood. Hypoxia is a condition of deficient oxygen in the tissues.

Pyrexia is the medical term for a fever (pyr/o = fire).

Rhinorrhea (-rrhea = discharge) is a discharge from the nose.

Shortness of breath is a term for breathlessness, or air hunger.

Sputum is the mucous that is coughed up from the lungs and expectorated through the mouth. If abnormal, it would be described in terms of its amount, color, and/or odor.

Thoracodynia (thorac/o = chest + -dynia = pain) is a term for chest pain.

Each of the following terms ends with the suffix –pnea, which means breathing.

Dyspnea is abnormal, difficult, or uncomfortable breathing.

Eupnea (eu- = good, normal) is good, normal breathing.

Apnea (a- = without) means a temporary lack of breathing. If it was permanent the patient would have expired!

Bradypnea (brady- = slow) is abnormally slow breathing.

Hyperpnea (hyper- = excessive) is excessively deep breathing. Hypopnea (hypo-=deficient) is extremely shallow breathing.

Orthopnea (orth/o = straight) is a condition of difficult breathing unless the patient is in an upright position.

Tachypnea is rapid, shallow breathing.

Friction sounds are those that are made by rubbing together of dry surfaces. A hiccup is a sound produced by the involuntary contraction of the diaphragm, followed by rapid closure of the glottis (the opening between the vocal cords). Rales (also called crackles) are discontinuous bubbling noises. Rhonchi are abnormal rumbling sounds caused by airways blocked by secretions or muscle contractions. Stridor is a high-pitched inspiratory sound from the larynx. It is a sign of an obstruction of the upper airway. Chest tympany is low-pitched resonant sounds heard in the chest. Wheezing is a whistling sound made during breathing.

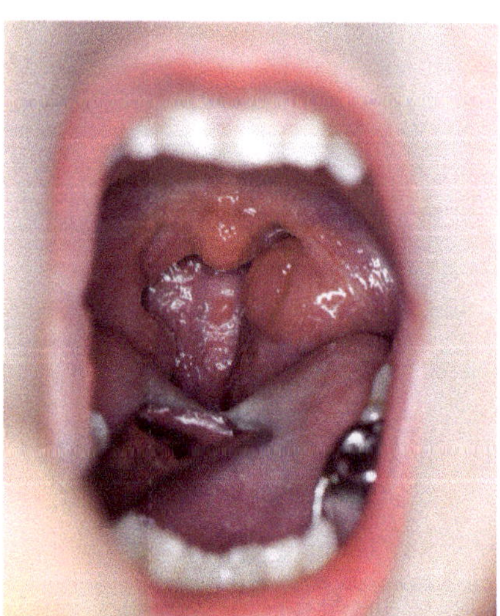
© Oleg Malyshev/Shutterstock.com

Coryza is a term for the common cold.

Croup is an acute viral infection of early childhood, marked by stridor caused by spasms of the larynx, trachea, and bronchi.

A deviated septum is a deflection of the wall between the nares that may obstruct the nasal passages. It may cause infection, sinusitis, shortness of breath, headache, or recurring epistaxis.

Epiglottitis is an inflammation of the epiglottis.

Laryngitis is an inflammation of the larynx.

Pharyngitis is an inflammation of the throat.

Asthma is a respiratory disorder that is characterized by recurring episodes of paroxysmal (sudden, episodic) dyspnea. Patients exhibit coughing, wheezing, and shortness of breath. If the attack is continuous, it is referred to as status asthmaticus, which may be fatal.

Bronchospasm (-spasm = sudden, involuntary contraction) is a sudden, involuntary contraction of the bronchi, as in an asthma attack.

Bronchiolitis is a viral inflammation of the bronchioles, most common in young children.

Bronchitis is an inflammation of the bronchi that may be acute or chronic.

Emphysema is an abnormal condition characterized by distension and destructive changes of the alveoli.

Acute respiratory failure is a sudden inability of the respiratory system to provide oxygen and/or remove carbon dioxide from the blood.

Cystic fibrosis is an inherited disorder of the exocrine glands of the lungs, resulting in abnormal, thick secretions of mucus.

Atelectasis is a collapse of the lung tissue or an entire lung. (a-= not + tel/o = complete + -ectasis = dilation)

Flail chest is a condition in which multiple rib fractures cause an instability in part of the chest wall. Because of this, the lung under the injured area contracts on inspiration and bulges out on expiration.

Influenza is the term for an infectious condition of the respiratory system caused by a virus. This is commonly called the flu. The avian (bird) flu is caused by the type A influenza virus.

Diphtheria is a bacterial respiratory disorder characterized by a sore throat, fever, and headache. It is one of the diseases for which a vaccination is available (DPT vaccine: diphtheria, pertussis, and tetanus).

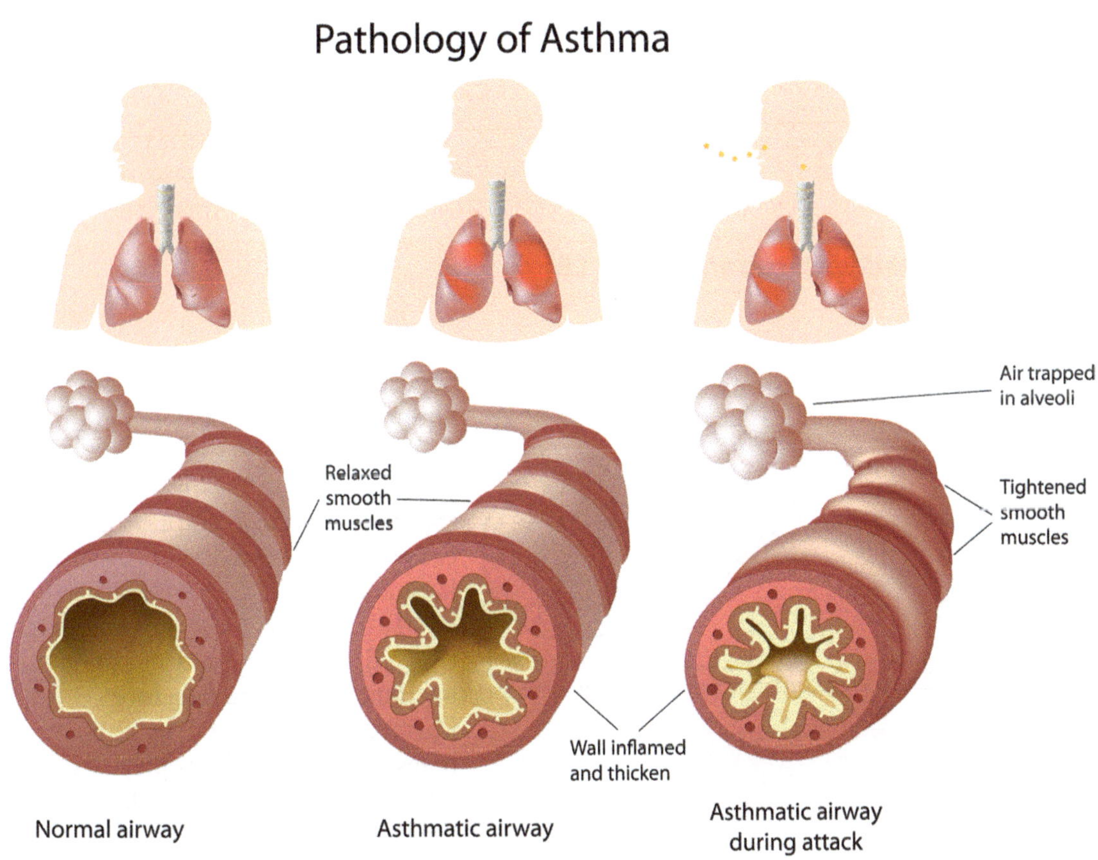

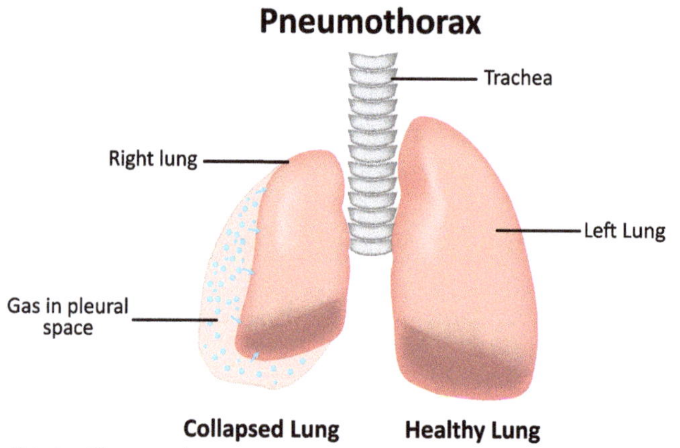

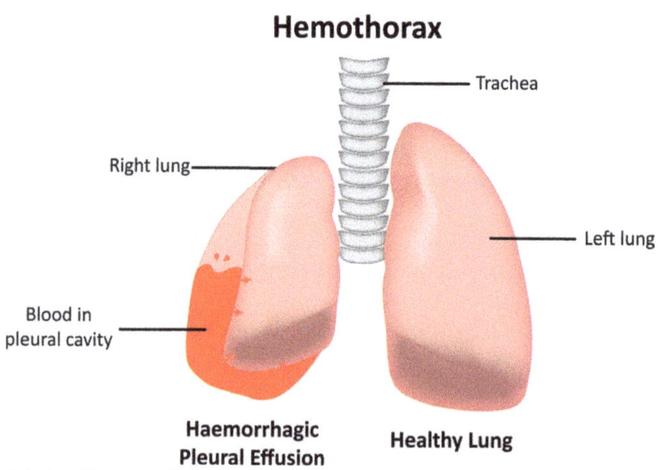

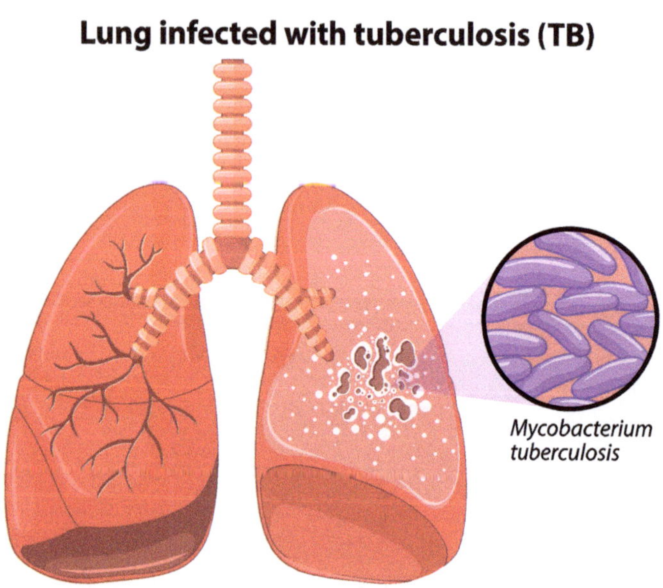

Pertussis, also called whooping cough, is a bacterial infection of the respiratory tract, characterized by a high-pitched "whoop." This is also avoidable via the DPT vaccine.

The suffix –thorax literally means the chest, but in the following terms, it refers to the pleural cavity.

Hemothorax is blood in the pleural cavity.

Pneumothorax (pneum/o = air) is air in the pleural cavity.

Pyothorax (py/o = pus) is pus in the pleural cavity.

Pneumonia is an inflammation of the lungs caused by a variety of pathogens. If infectious, it is termed pneumonia; if it is noninfectious, it is termed pneumonitis. Pneumonia is further named by the extent of the disease, for example, RML pneumonia is right median lobe pneumonia, whereas double pneumonia is an involvement of both lungs.

A pulmonary abscess is a localized accumulation of pus in the lungs.

Pulmonary edema is an accumulation of fluid in the lung tissue. This is often seen in congestive heart failure and is caused by the inability of the heart to pump blood.

Respiratory syncytial virus (RSV) is an acute respiratory disorder usually occurring in the lower respiratory tract in children and the upper respiratory tract in adults.

Severe acute respiratory syndrome (SARS) is a viral respiratory disorder caused by a coronavirus. It usually results in pneumonia.

Tuberculosis (TB) is a chronic infectious disorder caused by an acid-fast bacillus, *Mycobacterium tuberculosis*. It is normally transmitted by inhalation or ingestion of infected droplets. Multidrug-resistant TB (MDR TB) is fatal in 80% of the cases.

Auscultation is the act of listening to sounds within a patient's chest, whereas percussion is a tapping of the body walls. Don't confuse the abbreviation A&P with the same one that is used for anatomy and physiology! If no sounds are heard in the chest that would indicate fluid or exudates, the patient is said to be "clear to auscultation," abbreviated CTA.

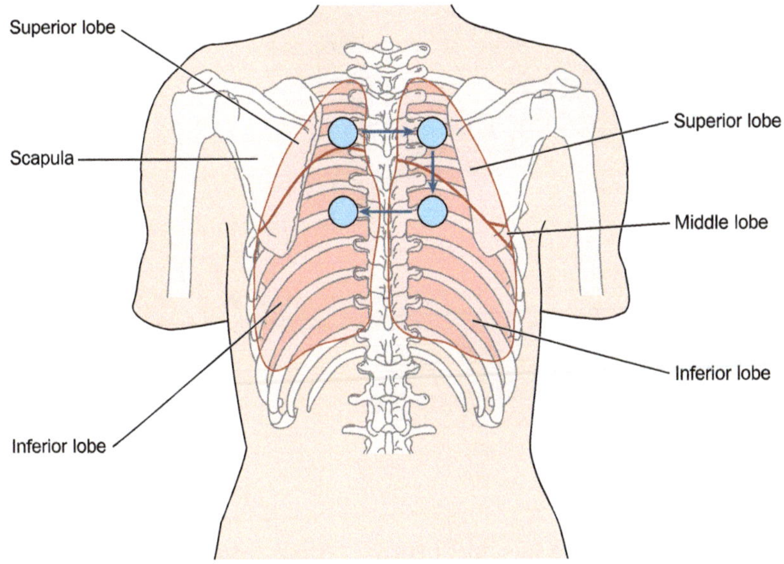

© Blamb/Shutterstock.com

Further examination of the chest by listening may be accomplished using a stethoscope (steth/o = chest). Note that the prefix -scope, which normally means *an instrument to view*, is used to indicate *an instrument to listen* in this one example.

All of the following are endoscopic procedures; that is, procedures that require an instrument to view (-scope) within (endo-) the body.

A bronchoscopy is the process of viewing the bronchial tubes.

A laryngoscopy is the process of viewing the interior of the larynx (the voice box).

Mediastinoscopy is the process of viewing the structures contained between the lungs.

A thoracoscopy is the process of viewing the entire chest cavity.

Arterial blood gases (ABG) is a blood test that measures the amount of oxygen and carbon dioxide in the blood. Note that this is one of the very few tests in which blood is taken from an artery instead of a vein.

Pulse oximetry (ox/i = oxygen + -metry = process of measurement) is a simple noninvasive test that is done to measure oxygen in arterial blood; it is done through the use of a clip-like device attached to either the earlobe or the fingertip.

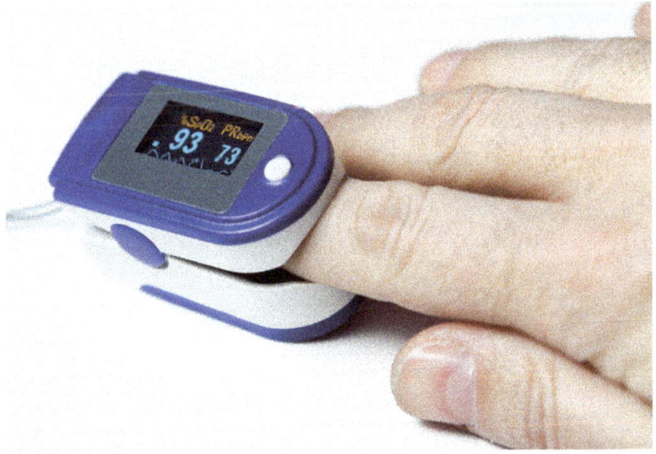

© Juan R. Velasco/Shutterstock.com

The Mantoux skin test is an intradermal (intra- = within) injection of purified protein derivative (PPD), which is done to detect the presence of tuberculosis antibodies.

The quantiferon-TB gold test is a definitive test to diagnose tuberculosis.

A sputum culture and sensitivity is the cultivation of microorganisms from sputum that has been collected from expectoration (ex- = out + pector/o = chest).

A throat culture is the cultivation of microorganisms from a throat swab to

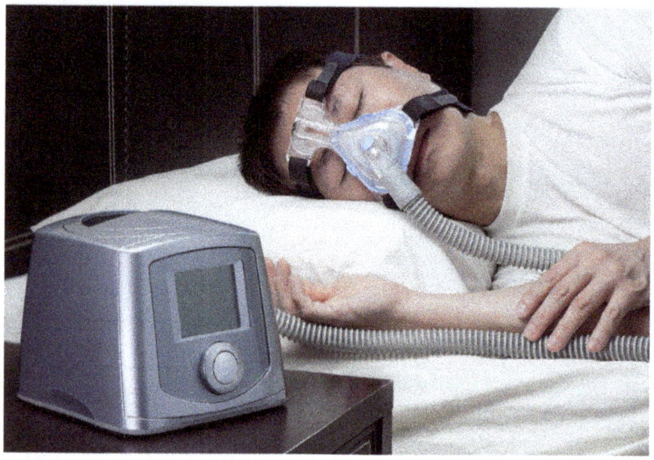

© Chalermpon Poungpeth/Shutterstock.com

determine the type of organism causing a suspected infection of the throat.

A sweat test is a method of evaluating the concentration of sodium and chloride in sweat as a means of diagnosing cystic fibrosis.

A ventilator is a mechanical device to provide oxygen through positive-pressure breathing. This is a respiratory therapy technique designed to deliver air at greater than atmospheric pressure to the lungs.

Continuous positive airway pressure (CPAP) is another method of delivery. Air can be delivered through a ventilator and endotracheal tubes or nasal cannulae, face masks, or hoods over the patient's head.

A nasal cannula (a set of pronged tubes inserted in the nostrils) is used to deliver a low level of oxygen.

A simple face mask is a plastic device that covers the nose and mouth and is used to deliver oxygen; a Venturi mask is similar but has a much larger tube that connects the oxygen source to the mask.

A rebreathing mask is used if higher oxygen levels are needed. This again is similar to a face mask but has one-way valve that allow for little or no rebreathing to take place so that the patient can have a richer continuous oxygen supply.

Endotracheal (endo- = within) intubation is the passage of a tube through the mouth into the trachea to ensure a patent (open) airway.

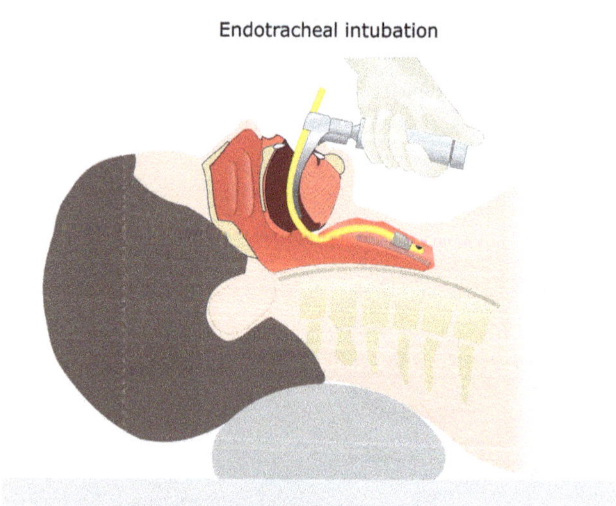

© ellepigrafica/Shutterstock.com

Thoracentesis (also called a pleurocentesis) is the surgical puncture of the pleura to aspirate fluid.

A thoracotomy is an incision in the chest as a means of approach for surgery.

A sinusotomy is an incision in a sinus.

A tracheotomy is an incision in the trachea, whereas a tracheostomy is a new opening through which an indwelling tube may be inserted temporarily or permanently. The tracheotomy is usually an emergency procedure to gain access to the airway.

The respiratory system is as complex as the circulatory system. Without this system our body cannot function. Our ability to understand and intervene in the respiratory system is necessary for us to provide great patient care.

CHAPTER 9

Nervous

The nervous system is typically described as having two divisions: the central nervous system (CNS) and the peripheral nervous system (PNS). The CNS is made up of the brain and spinal cord. It is enclosed by bones of the skull and spinal column. The PNS is made up of nerves and neural tissue branching all over the body from 12 pair of cranial nerves and 31 pair of spinal nerves.

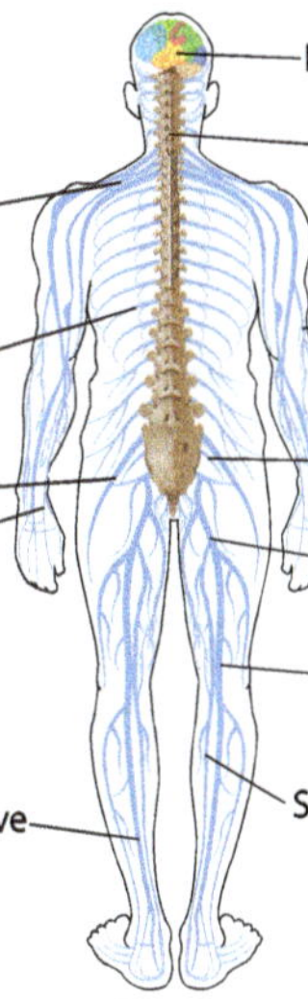

© snapgalleria/Shutterstock.com

The PNS includes the nerves that travel to the point of sensation and those that carry the sensation back to the brain. These are termed the efferent (or motor) nerves and the afferent (or sensory) nerves.

Somatic nerves collect information from and return instructions to the skin, muscles, and joints. The autonomic nerves are mostly involuntary and collect information from the internal environment in the body. The information is sent to the CNS, where in return, motor impulses are sent to involuntary muscles in the heart, glands, and organs.

Remember that efferent means to carry away and afferent means to carry toward. In the nervous system, these terms are used to refer to away from and toward the brain.

The central nervous system consists of the brain and the spinal cord.

The brain is divided into four sections: the cerebrum, the cerebellum, the diencephalon, and the brainstem.

Myel/o means bone marrow or spinal cord; memorization and context will be the student's only methods to determine which is which.

The cerebrum, the largest part of the brain, is divided into two hemispheres. It is responsible for thinking, reasoning, and memory. The surfaces are covered with gray matter called the cerebral cortex, which is folded into sulci (valleys) and gyri (ridges). The cerebrum has four lobes that have varying functions.

Frontal lobe: speech and voluntary motor movement on the contralateral side of the body.
Temporal lobe: auditory and olfactory functions.
Parietal lobe: sensations of touch and taste.
Occipital lobe: vision.

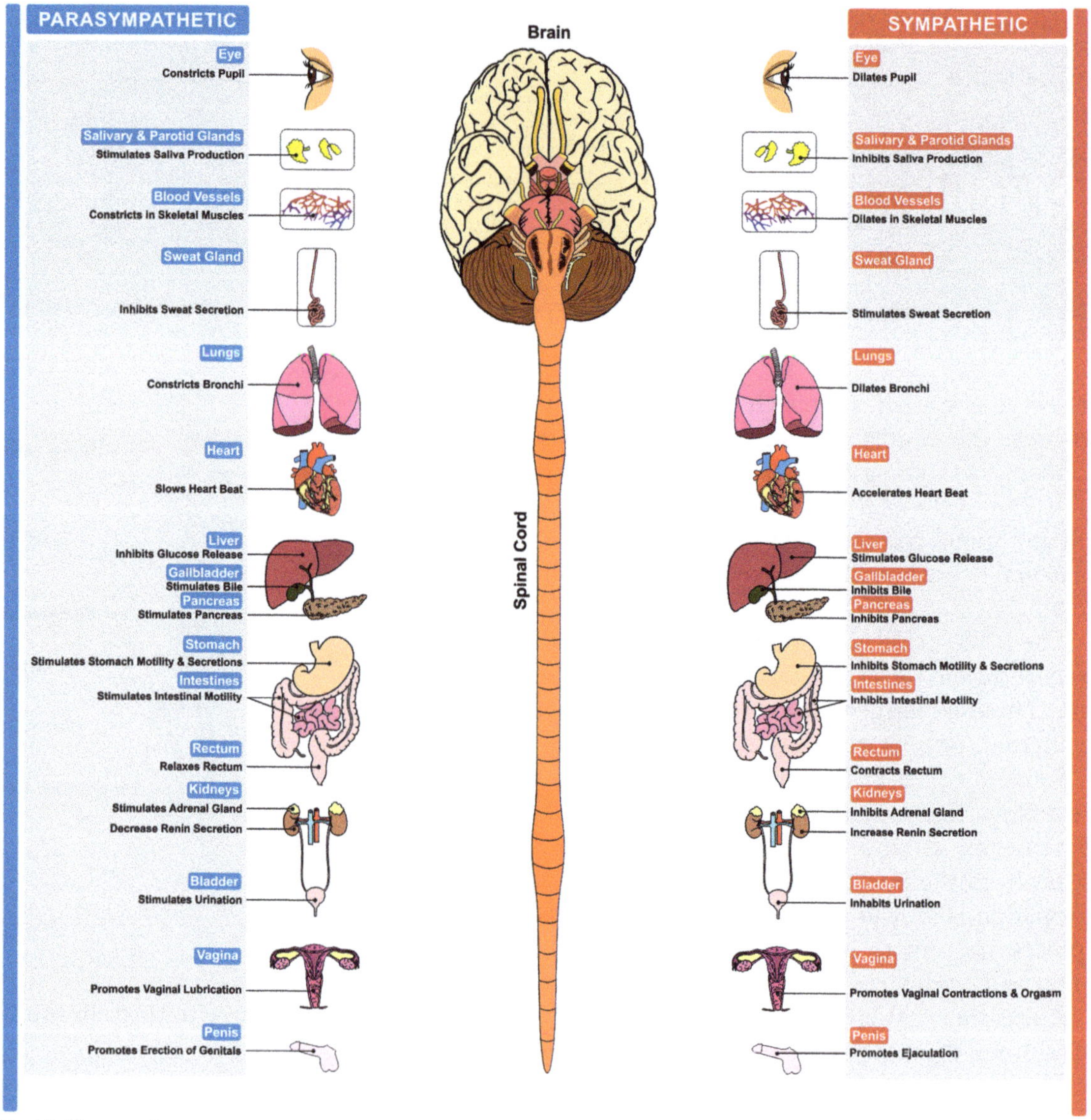

© udaix/Shutterstock.com

The cerebellum is inferior to the occipital lobe of the cerebrum, it coordinates voluntary movement but is involuntary in function.

The diencephalon composed of the thalamus and the hypothalamus. The thalamus relays sensory information (except for the sense of smell) and translates it into sensations of pain, temperature, and touch. The hypothalamus activates, integrates, and controls the peripheral autonomic nervous system, along with temperature, sleep, and appetite.

The brainstem connects the cerebral hemispheres to the spinal cord. It is composed of the midbrain, pons, and medulla oblongata. The midbrain connects the pons and cerebellum with the cerebral hemispheres. It is the site of reflex centers for eye and head movements in response to visual and auditory stimuli. The pons serves as a bridge between the medulla oblongata and the cerebrum. The medulla oblongata regulates heart rate, blood pressure, and breathing.

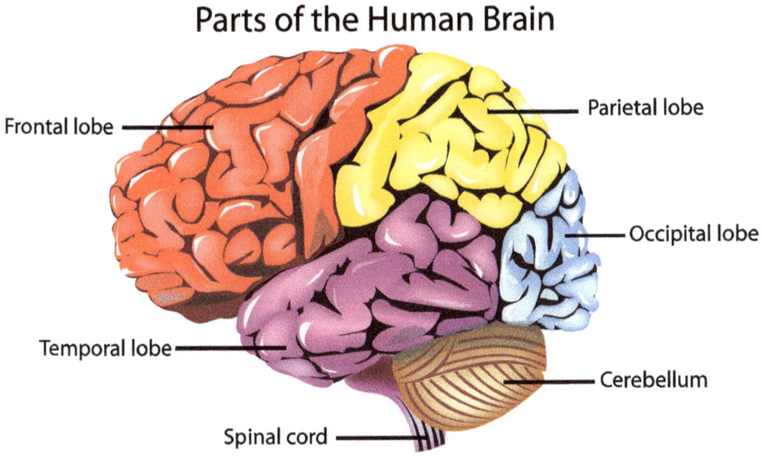

© GraphicsRF/Shutterstock.com

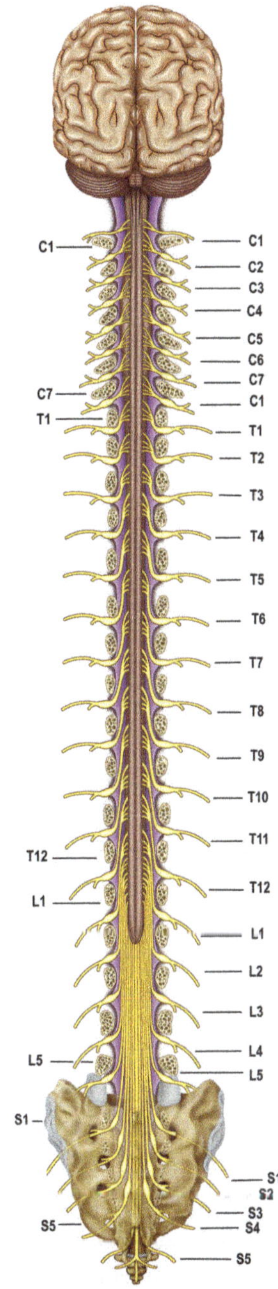

© Alexilusmedical/Shutterstock.com

The spinal cord extends from the medulla oblongata to the first lumbar vertebra, where it divides into the structure called the cauda equina, which is a Latin term meaning horse tail.

Locate the nerve roots in the illustration and name the combining forms.

The bony vertebrae surrounding the spinal cord protect it, along with the coating of the CNS called the meninges. The spinal cord is composed of gray matter (the cell bodies of motor neurons) and white matter (the myelin-covered axons or nerve fibers that extend from the nerve cell bodies). The 31 pairs of spinal nerves emerge from the spinal cord at the nerve roots.

The meninges are arranged in three layers that are separated by spaces.

The dura mater is the tough outer covering of the meninges. Dura mater literally means "hard mother."

The space underneath the dura mater is the subdural space.

The next layer is the arachnoid membrane. It is a thin, delicate membrane that takes its name from its spidery appearance (arachn/o = spider + -oid = resembling). The space underneath is called the subarachnoid space, which contains the cerebrospinal fluid. This fluid is continuous with the ventricles of the brain. The final layer is the pia mater (literally the "soft mother"), which is a thin, vascular membrane.

The peripheral nervous system is divided into 12 pairs of cranial nerves that conduct impulses between the brain and head, neck, thoracic and abdominal areas, and 31 pairs of spinal nerves that provide innervation to the rest of the body. Cranial nerves are named by their number and their function or distribution. For example, the **vestibulocochlear nerve** (also known as the **auditory** or **acoustic nerve**) is the eighth of the twelve cranial nerves. Spinal nerves are named by their location (cervical, thoracic, lumbar, sacral, and cocygeal) and by their number.

A plexus is a network of nerve fibers from several spinal nerves.

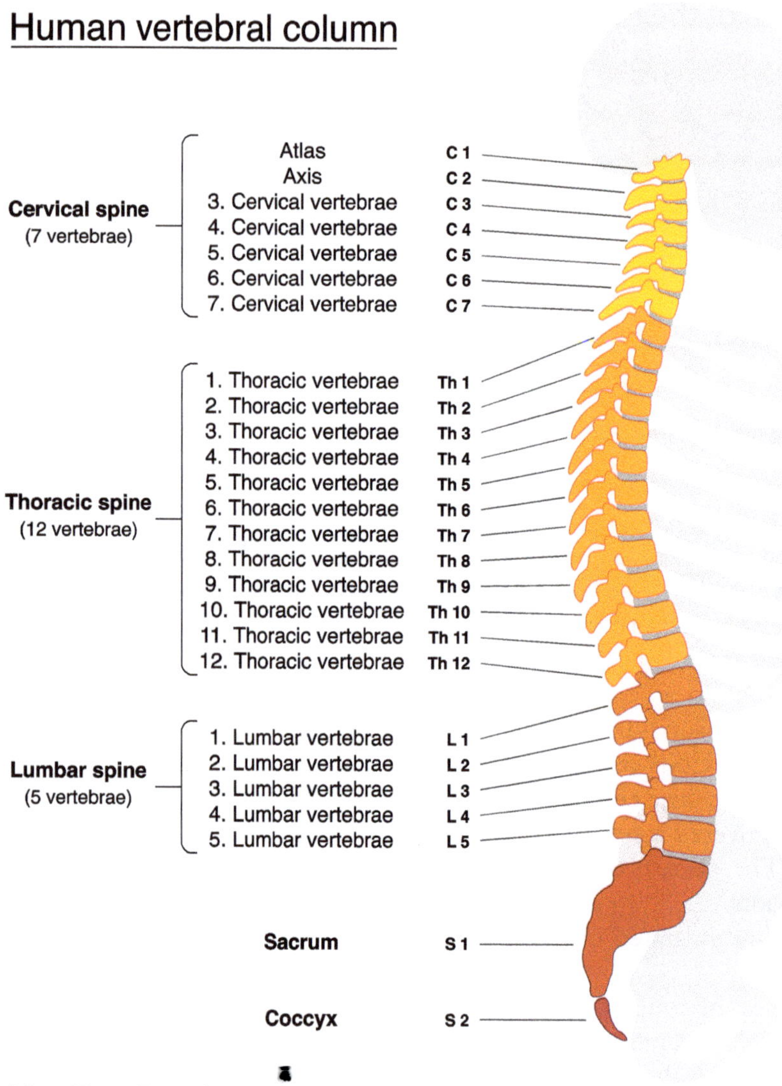

A dermatome is the skin surface area supplied by a single afferent spinal nerve. Use the diagram to show how these areas can be specifically mapped. Patients with shingles show similar patterns as a specific peripheral nerve is affected with the disorder. Be careful! The term *dermatome* can be used to describe an instrument that cuts thin slices of skin for grafting, and the term also signifies a mesodermal layer in early development, which becomes the dermal layers of the skin.

The autonomic nervous system consists of nerves that regulate involuntary function (cardiac and smooth muscles). The motor portion of this system is further divided into the sympathetic and parasympathetic nervous systems. Sympathetic nervous system: fight or flight. It helps individual respond to stressful situations. Heart rate and blood pressure increase, digestion slows, and sweat and adrenal glands increase secretion. Parasympathetic nervous system: rest and digest. It helps balance the effect of the sympathetic response. Heart and blood pressure decrease, digestion increases, and adrenal and sweat gland activities decrease.

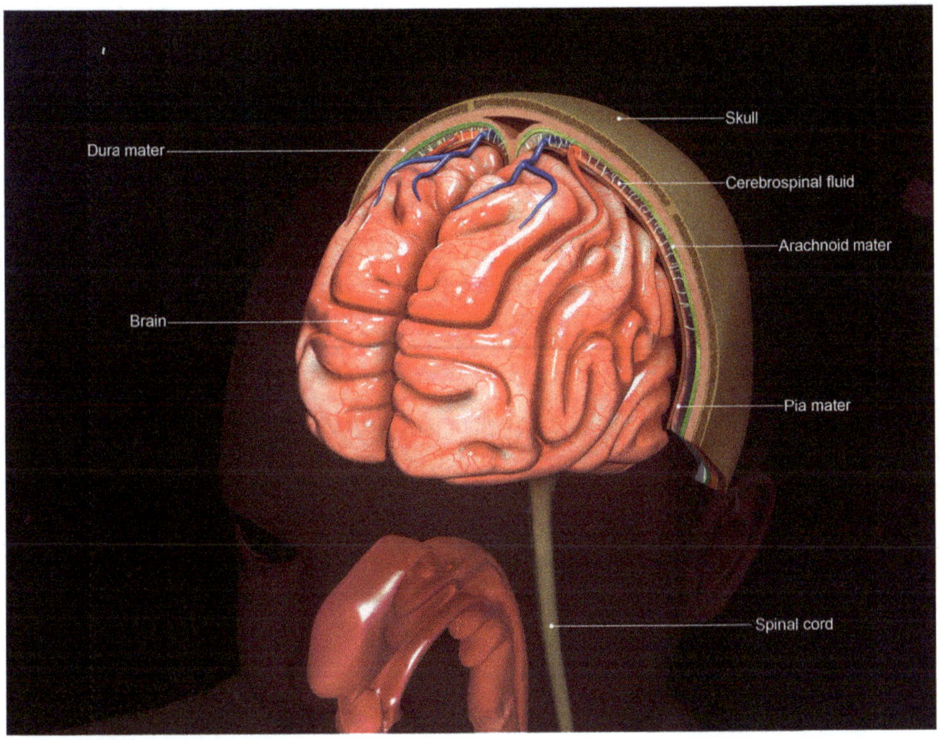

Cerebral palsy is a motor function disorder resulting from a permanent, nonprogressive brain defect or lesion caused perinatally (peri- = surround + nat/o = birth). Neural deficits may include paralysis, ataxia, athetosis (slow, writhing movements of the extremities), seizure, and/or impairment of sensory functions.

Huntington chorea is an inherited disorder that manifests itself in adulthood as a progressive loss of neural control, uncontrollable jerking movements, and dementia.

Hydrocephalus (hydr/o = water + -cephalus = head) is a condition of an abnormal accumulation of fluid in the ventricles of the brain; it may or may not result in mental retardation. Although usually diagnosed in babies, it may also occur in adults as a result of stroke, trauma, or infection.

Spina bifida (bi- = two + -fida = split) is a condition in which the spinal column has an abnormal opening that allows protrusion of the meninges and/or the spinal cord. This is termed a meningocele (mening/o = meninges + -cele = herniation) or meningomyelocele (mening/o = meninges + myel/o = spinal cord + -cele = herniation).

Tay-Sachs disease is an inherited disease that occurs mainly in the people of Eastern European Jewish origin; it is caused by an enzyme deficiency that results in CNS deterioration.

A coma is a deep, prolonged unconsciousness from which the patient cannot be aroused; it is usually the result of a head injury, neurologic disease, acute hydrocephalus, intoxication, or metabolic abnormalities.

A concussion is a serious head injury characterized by one or more of the following: loss of consciousness, amnesia, seizures, or a change in mental status.

A cerebral contusion is a head injury of sufficient force to bruise the brain. Bruising of the brain often involves the brain surface and causes extravasation of blood without rupture of the pia-arachnoid membranes. It is often associated with a concussion.

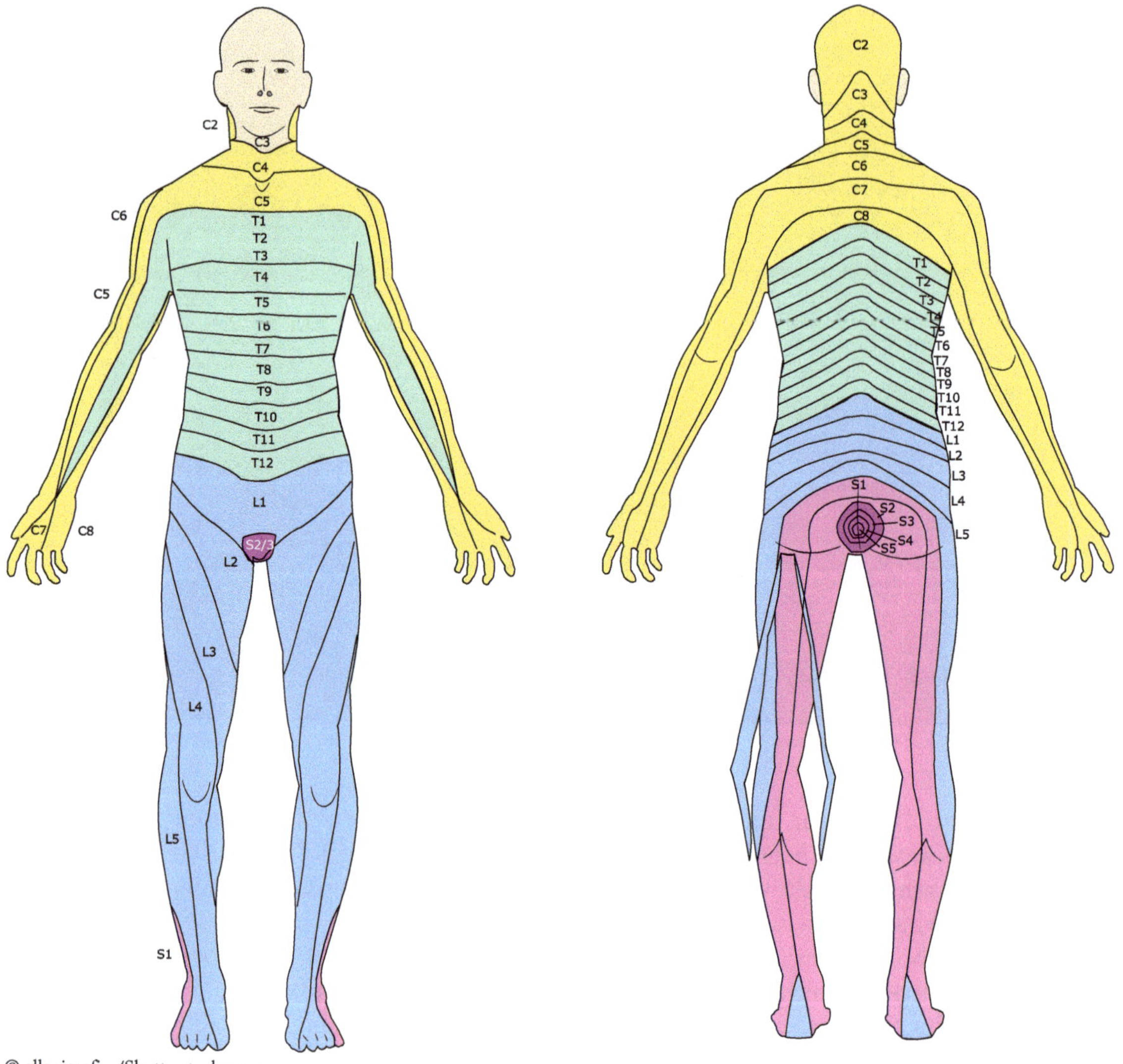

© ellepigrafica/Shutterstock.com

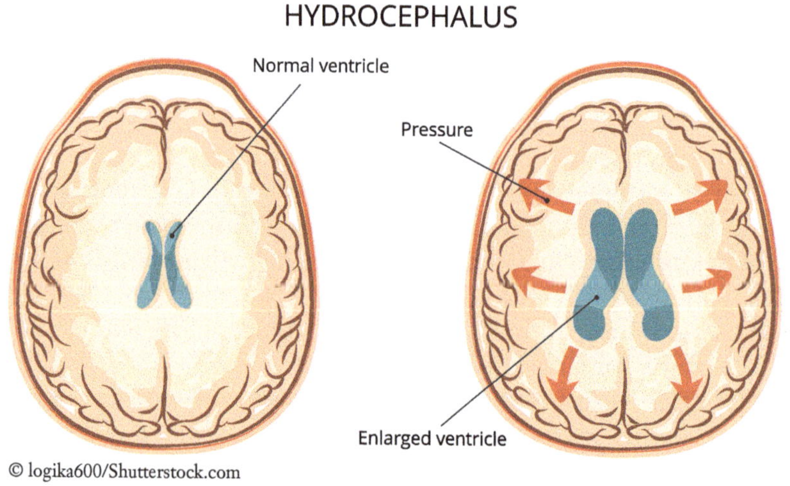

© logika600/Shutterstock.com

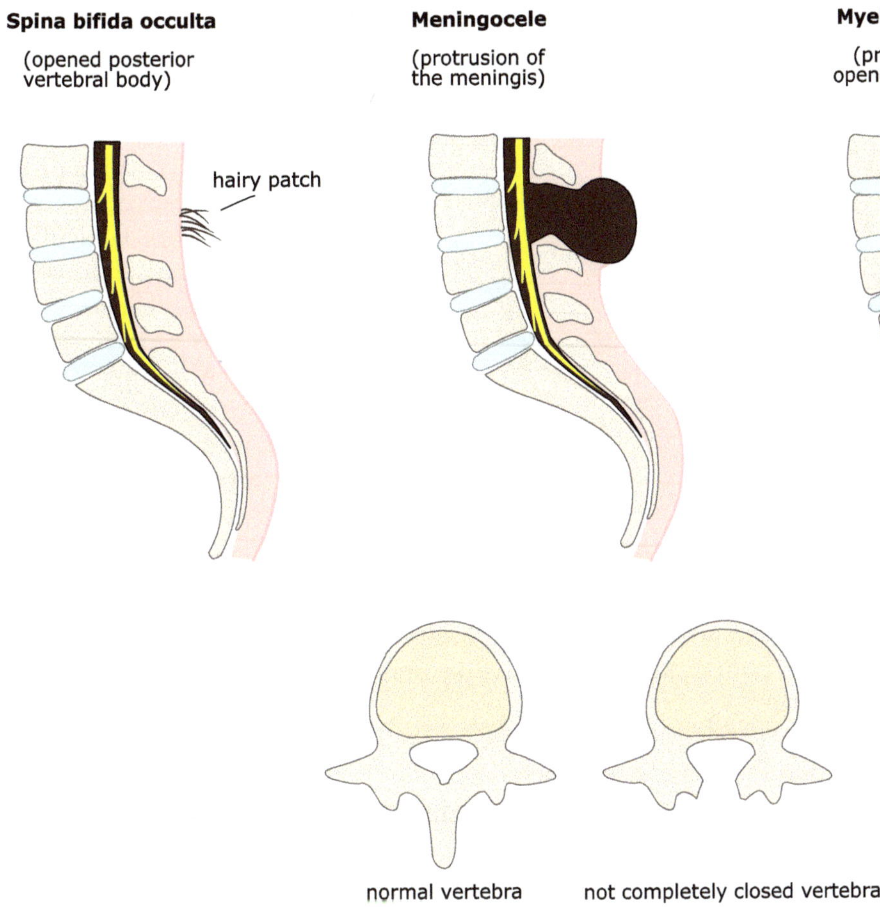

© ellepigrafica/Shutterstock.com

A hematoma (hemat/o = blood + -oma = mass) is a localized collection of blood, usually clotted, in an organ, tissue, or space, due to a break in the wall of a blood vessel. Use the diagrams to show the different types of hematomas.

A herniated intervertebral disk (HIVD) (inter- = between + vertebr/o = vertebra + -al = pertaining to) is a displacement of an intervertebral disk so that it presses on a nerve, causing pain and/or numbness.

Alzheimer's disease (not old timer disease!) is a progressive, neurodegenerative disease in which patients exhibit an impairment of cognitive functioning. The cause of the disease is unknown. Alzheimer's disease is the most common cause of dementia. This image shows that a brain affected by Alzheimer's disease (top) is smaller with narrow gyri (ridges) and widened sulci (valleys). The lower brain is normal.

Amyotrophic lateral sclerosis (a- = no + my/o = muscle + troph/o = development + -ic = pertaining to, later/o = side + -al = pertaining to, sclerosis = abnormal condition of hardening) is a degenerative, fatal disease of the motor neurons, in which patients exhibit progressive muscle weakness and atrophy. Also called Lou Gehrig disease after Lou Gehrig, a talented baseball player with the disorder.

Guillain-Barré syndrome is an autoimmune disorder of acute polyneuritis producing profound myasthenia (muscle weakness) that may lead to paralysis.

Multiple sclerosis (MS) is a neurodegenerative disease characterized by destruction of the myelin sheaths on the CNS neurons (demyelination) and their abnormal replacement by the gradual accumulation of hardened plaques. The disease may be progressive or characterized by remissions and

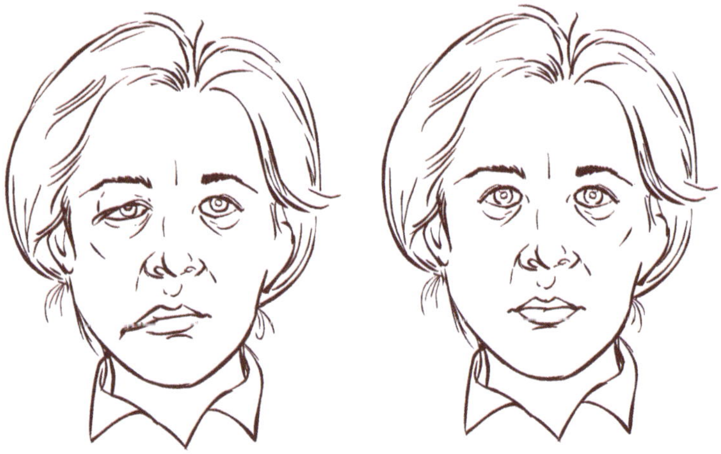

© corbac40/Shutterstock.com

relapses. The cause is unknown. Be careful! MS stands for both musculoskeletal system, mitral stenosis, and multiple sclerosis.

Parkinson's disease is a progressive neurodegenerative disease characterized by tremors, fasciculations, slow shuffling gait, hypokinesia, dysphasia, and dysphagia.

Bell palsy is a paralysis of the facial nerve. Although the cause is unknown, the condition usually resolves on its own in 6 months.

Epilepsy (epi- = above + -lepsy = seizure) is a group of disorders characterized by some or all of the following: recurrent seizures, sensory disturbances, abnormal behavior, and/or loss of consciousness. Types of seizures include:

Tonic clonic (grand mal): temporary loss of consciousness and severe muscle spasms.
Absence (petit mal): loss of consciousness exhibited by unresponsiveness for short periods without muscle involvement.
Status epilepticus: intense, unrelenting, life-threatening seizures.
Pseudoseizures (pseudo- = false) are false seizures.
Causes may be due to trauma, tumor, intoxication, chemical imbalance, or vascular disturbances.

Narcolepsy (narc/o = sleep + -lepsy = seizure) is a disorder characterized by sudden attacks of sleep.

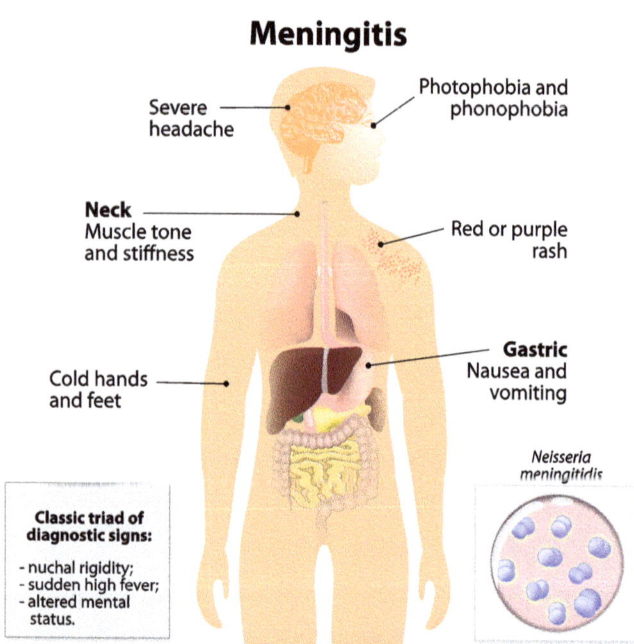

© Designua/Shutterstock.com

Tourette syndrome is an abnormal condition characterized by facial grimaces, tics, involuntary arm and shoulder movements, and involuntary vocalizations including coprolalia (copr/o = feces + -lalia = condition of babbling). Coprolalia is vulgar, obscene, or sacrilegious language.

Encephalitis (encephal/o = brain + -itis = inflammation) is an inflammation of the brain, most frequently caused by a virus transmitted by the bite of an infected mosquito.

Meningitis (mening/o = meninges + -itis = inflammation) is any infection or inflammation of the membranes covering the brain and spinal cord, most commonly due to viral infection. The more severe strains are bacterial or fungal in nature. Symptoms include stiff neck and sudden high fever.

Neuritis (neur/o = nerve + -itis = inflammation) is an inflammation of the nerves.

Poliomyelitis (polio- = gray + myel/o = spinal cord + -itis = inflammation) is an inflammation of the gray matter of the spinal cord caused by a poliovirus. Some forms cause paralysis.

Polyneuritis (poly- = many + neur/o = nerve + -itis = inflammation) is an inflammation of several peripheral nerves.

Radiculitis (radicul/o = nerve root + -itis = inflammation) is an inflammation of the root of a spinal nerve.

Sciatica is an inflammation of the sciatic nerve. Symptoms include pain and tenderness along the path of the nerve through the thigh and leg.

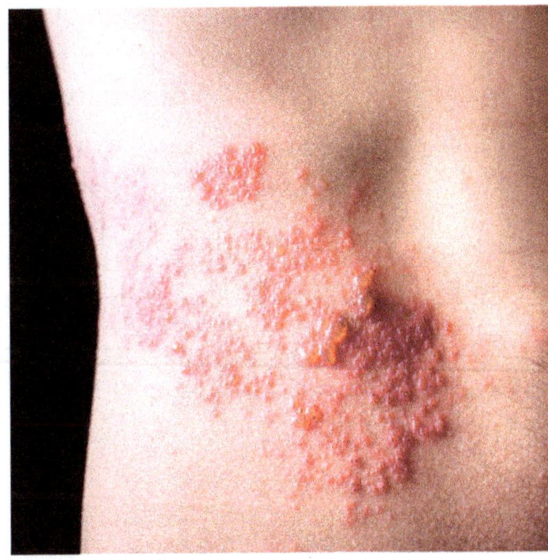

Shingles is an acute infection caused by the latent varicella zoster virus (chicken pox), characterized by the development of vesicular skin eruption underlying the route of cranial or spinal nerves. Also called herpes zoster.

A cerebrovascular (cerebr/o = cerebrum + vascul/o = vessel + -ar = pertaining to) accident (CVA) is ischemia (a lack of blood flow) of cerebral tissue due to an occlusion (blockage) from a thrombus or embolus, or as a result of a cerebral hemorrhage. Results of a stroke depend on the duration and location of the ischemia. These sequelae may include paralysis, weakness, speech defects, sensory changes that last longer than 24 hours, and death. Other names for a CVA are stroke, brain attack, and cerebral infarction (an infarction means tissue death).

A migraine is a headache of vascular origin. It may be classified as migraine with aura (premonitions) or migraine without aura.

A transient ischemic attack (ischem/o = to hold back + -ic = pertaining to) has the same mechanisms as those of a CVA, but the sequelae resolve and disappear within 24 hours. It is commonly referred to as a ministroke.

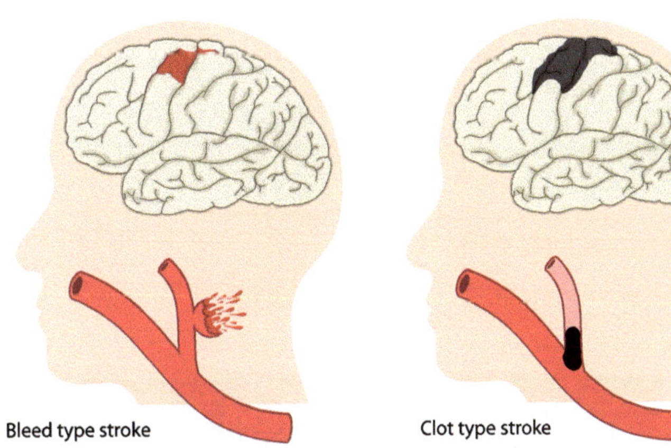

Paralytic conditions are generally described by the suffixes –plegia meaning paralysis (the loss of muscle function, sensation, or both) and –paresis, meaning a slight paralysis. These conditions are usually further described by the area of the body affected.

Diplegia (di- = two) is a paralysis of the same body part on both sides of the body.
Hemiplegia (hemi- = half) is a paralysis on the left or right side of the body.
Monoplegia (mono- = one) is a paralysis of one limb on the left or right side of the body.
Paraplegia (para- = abnormal) is paralysis of the lower limbs and trunk.
Quadriplegia (quadri- = four) is paralysis of arms, legs, and trunk.

A brain scan is a nuclear medicine procedure involving intravenous injection of radioisotopes to localize and identify intracranial masses, lesions, tumors, or infarcts. The photography is done by a scintillator or scanner.

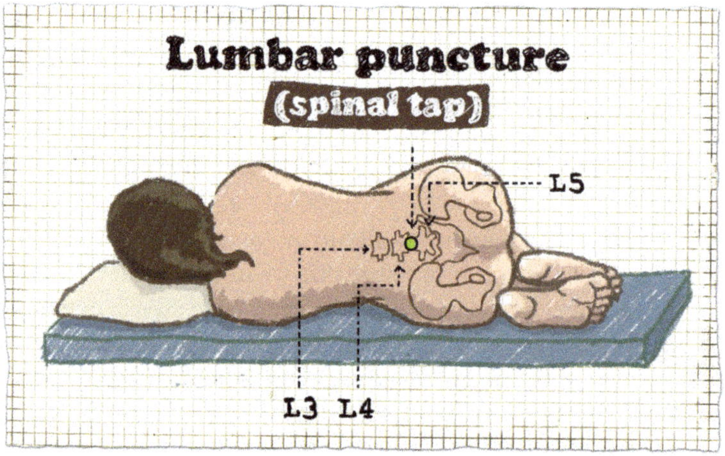

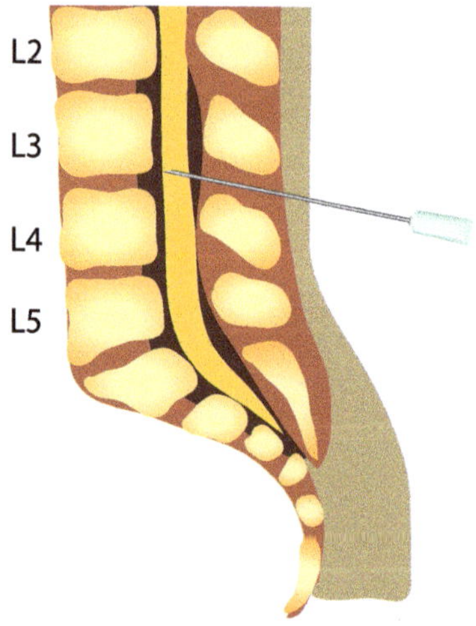

Lumbar Puncture

Cerebral angiography (angi/o = vessel + -graphy = process of recording) is an x-ray of the cerebral arteries, including the internal carotids, taken after the injection of a contrast medium. The procedure is also termed a cerebral arteriography.

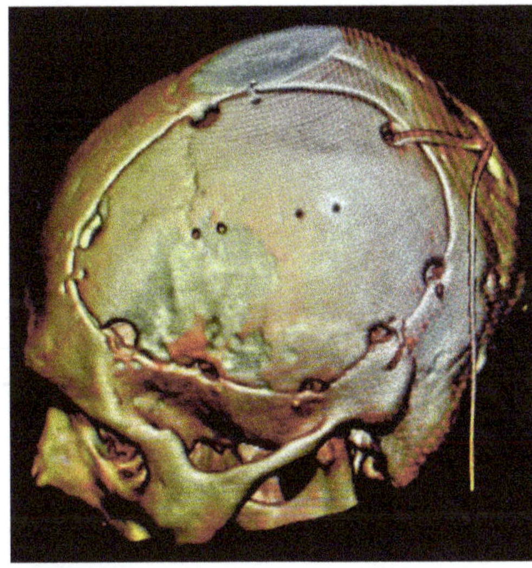

Computed tomography is the transverse sections of the central nervous system that are imaged, sometimes after the injection of a contrast medium (unless there is suspected bleeding). It is used to diagnose strokes, edema, tumors, and hemorrhage resulting from trauma.

A lumbar puncture (lumb/o = lower back + -ar = pertaining to) is a procedure to aspirate cerebrospinal fluid (CSF) from the lumbar subarachnoid space. A needle is inserted between two lumbar vertebrae to withdraw the fluid for diagnostic purposes. It is also called a spinal tap.

A craniotomy (crani/o = skull, cranium + -tomy = incision) is an incision into the skull as a surgical approach or to relieve intracranial pressure; it is also called trephination.

The nervous system is, in my opinion, the most complex system in the body. The body's ability to send electrical signals back and forth from specific areas in your body to your brain and back is remarkable. As healthcare providers, we must understand that nervous system and should be able to differentiate between the different processes and functions of the brain and spinal cord.

Chapter 10

Urinary

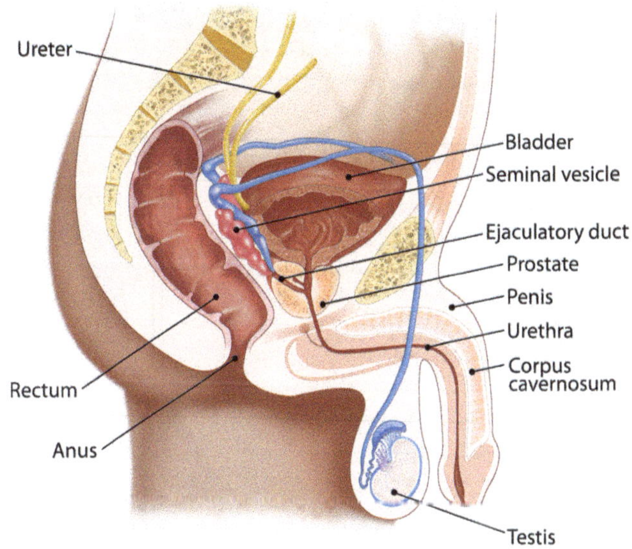

© kocakayaali/Shutterstock.com

The urinary system consists of two kidneys, two ureters, one bladder, and one urethra. This system goes by several different names: excretory, genitourinary, or urogenital systems, and is the organ that produces, stores, and eliminates urine. The primary functions of the urinary system are to extract wastes from the bloodstream, convert them to urine, transport the urine from the kidneys to the bladder, and eliminate it from the body. These vital functions help the body maintain homeostasis. home/o = same + -stasis = stopping, controlling. Homeostasis is a steady state, the process that the kidneys help maintain water balance in our bodies.

Obviously, the male and female urinary systems are very similar. Take a look at the length of the urethra in each. As the female urethra is so much shorter, infections (such as bladder infections) are much more common in women because the pathogens have less distance to travel to the bladder.

Each of these terms is used with regular frequency, so be flexible in your understanding of what each of the terms for "the process of releasing urine" means.

Urination—release of urine
Micturition—release of urine
Voiding—release of urine

During the day, the average person urinates about five times, usually 1.5 liters total.

Remember that stromal tissue is a supportive tissue. It doesn't do the work of the system, but it's necessary to help the parenchymal tissue (the kidneys) to carry out its work.

The ureters are the tubes that carry urine from the kidneys to the bladder. Again, these are paired, so the standard issue is two ureters. The combining form is ureter/o.

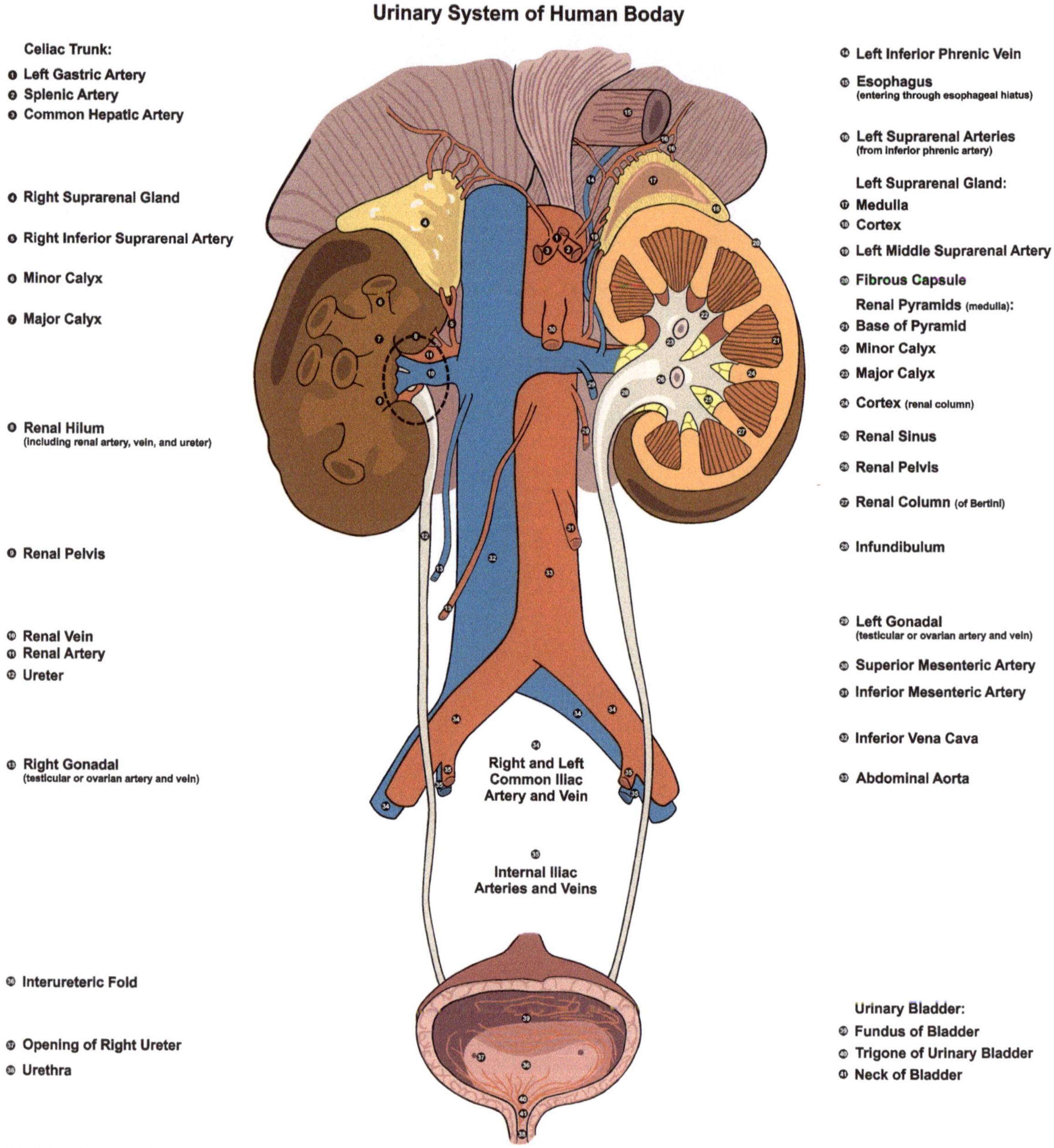

The urinary bladder is the sac that stores the urine until it is ready to be excreted. Note that the combining form that is commonly used for the urinary bladder is "cyst/o," which also means a "sac." The other combining form for the urinary bladder is vesic/o. You will see it being used in some of the terms later in the lecture. This also has a secondary meaning of "sac," and you may notice that in the integumentary chapter, we use the term "vesicle" to describe a blister. Makes sense! It's literally a "little sac."

Within the urinary bladder is an area that has a special name: the trigone. See the "tri-" at the beginning? Tri- means three. It gets its name from the two areas where the ureters join the bladder and the urethra exits. The combining form is trigon/o.

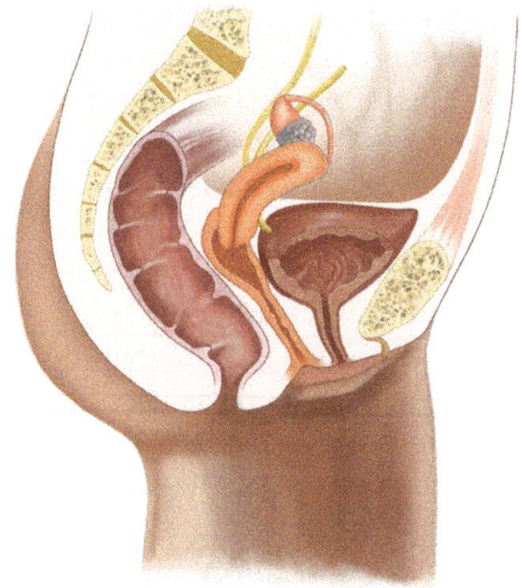

© kocakayaali/Shutterstock.com

Last, but not least, is the urethra. It is the tube that conducts urine from the bladder out of the body. The combining form for the urethra is urethr/o. Be careful not to confuse ureter/o with urethr/o. Remember that there are two of the first and one of the second.

The opening of the urethra is the urinary meatus. Pronunciation alert! That is mee ATE us. Obviously an opening to the urethra is important; we will discuss a term for abnormalities of this opening.

There are two kidneys, located in the retroperitoneal cavity. Each kidney is about the size of an individual's fist.

The cortex is the outer layer of the kidney, while the medulla is the middle part of the kidney. Both of these terms, cortex and medulla, are general terms and are also used to describe structures in other organs.

The calyces (s. calix/calyx) are part of the renal pelvis. **Be Careful! Calic/o** and **cali/o** are the combining forms for the calyx, but **calc/o** is the combining form for calcium.

Remember that a sign is an objective finding: it can be observed or measured. A symptom is a subjective impression and is experienced by the patient.

Albuminuria is a condition of protein in the urine. Albumin/o = protein + -uria = urinary condition. Albuminuria and proteinuria are synonyms.

Azoturia is a condition of excessive nitrogenous compounds in the urine. Azot/o = nitrogen + -uria = urinary condition.

Bacteriuria is a condition of bacteria in the urine. Bacteri/o = bacteria + -uria = urinary condition.

Glycosuria is a condition of sugar in the urine. Glycos/o = sugar + -uria = urinary condition.

Hematuria is a condition of blood in the urine. Hemat/o = blood + -uria = urinary condition.

Pyuria is a condition of pus in the urine. Py/o = pus + -uria = urinary condition. Be careful! **Py/o** means pus and **pyel/o** means renal pelvis. A dilation of the renal pelvis caused by an accumulation of pus would be pyopyelectasis.

Anuria is a condition of no urination. An- = no, not, without + -uria = urinary condition.

Dysuria is a condition of difficult or painful urination. Dys- = bad, difficult, painful + -uria = urinary condition.

Nocturia is a condition of (excessive) urination at night. Noct/i = night + -uria = urinary condition. It is not normal to get up several times a night to visit the bathroom, hence this term if that occurs. However, if an individual decides to drink a liter of soda right before going to bed and THEN needs to get up to urinate throughout the night, the appropriate term would be dumb, not nocturia.

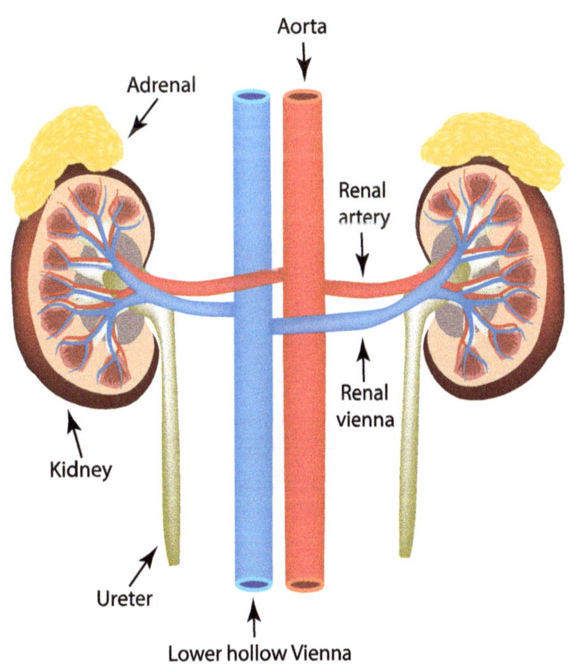

© Timonina/Shutterstock.com

Oliguria is a condition of scanty urination. Olig/o = scanty, few + -uria = urinary condition. This is a symptom of urinating only a small amount.

Finally, polyuria is excessive or profuse urination. Poly- = profuse, excessive + -uria = urinary condition.

Diuresis is a condition of increased formation and excretion of urine. It is a contraction of dia- = through, complete + ur/o = urine + -esis = state of. Diuretics can cause this symptom; some of the common ones that you may be familiar with are caffeine and alcohol.

Enuresis is commonly known as "bedwetting." If we switch the prefix on diuresis to "en-," which means "in," you can see that it is the "state of being in urine," which is precisely what would happen if one wet his or her bed. Technically, enuresis is named nocturnal (for night time occurrences) and diurnal (for daytime occurrences).

The term *polydipsia* means excessive thirst. Poly- = profuse, excessive + -dipsia = condition of thirst. What symptom do you think polydipsia could lead to? (polyuria)

Urinary incontinence is the inability to hold urine. Stress incontinence is the inability to hold urine with increased abdominal pressure, for example, when sneezing, coughing, laughing, or lifting.

Urinary retention is the inability to release urine.

Urgency is the need to urinate immediately

Particular types of UTIs are named for the organs that are involved; for example, bladder infections are termed *cystitis* (cyst/o = bladder).

Polycystic kidney disease is an inherited condition of bilateral (pertaining to the kidney on both sides) enlargement of the kidneys due to the development of multiple fluid-filled cysts. Poly- = many + cyst/o = sac + -ic = pertaining to.

Urolithiasis is the presence of stones within the urinary tract. Ur/o (urinary system) + lith/o (stones) + -iasis (condition, presence of). These stones can be associated with a particular structure, for example, nephrolithiasis (kidney stones), or described generally to be within the urinary system.

Nephrolithiasis is the presence of stones in the kidney. Nephr/o (kidney) + lith/o (stones) + -iasis (presence of).

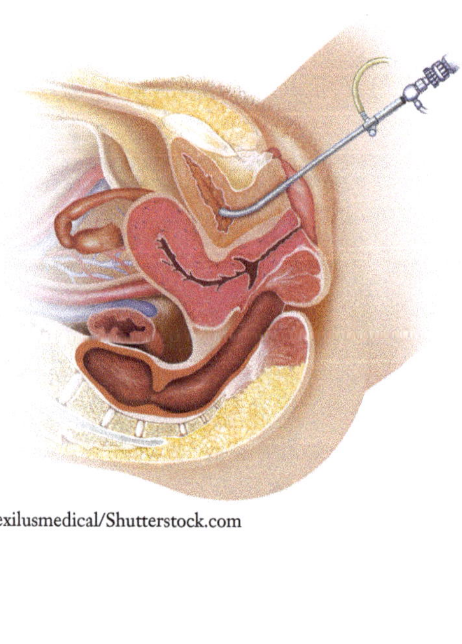

Renal colic is the severe pain that is often associated with kidney stones that become lodged in a ureter. The term *colic* is often associated with pain.

When kidneys can no longer perform their function of removing wastes from the blood, it is termed renal failure. This can be a sudden inability due to trauma, injury, or an obstruction, and is then termed acute renal failure (ARF). If it is ongoing, it is termed chronic kidney disease (formerly called chronic renal failure) and is measured in stages of increasing severity (1 being the lowest and 5 being complete kidney failure).

The appearance of urine is judged by its color–straw colored or light amber is considered normal; its quantity—normal excretion is 1.5 liters per day; and its specific gravity (SG), which is a measure of how concentrated it is. The normal reading is 1.015–1.025, slightly denser than the weight of water.

If the color is too light, it may indicate diabetes insipidus. If it is too dark, it may indicate dehydration, drugs, or liver disease.

If the quantity is too profuse, it may indicate diabetes insipidus or other diseases that cause diuresis. If it is too little, it may indicate dehydration, blockages, or strictures.

If the specific gravity is lower than normal, it may indicate diabetes or kidney damage.

Neither pus not bacteria should be present in the urine. Both of these would indicate an infection. A finding of bacteria may indicate a UTI, while pus could indicate pyelonephritis. Be careful! Don't mix up py/o meaning pus with pyel/o, meaning renal pelvis.

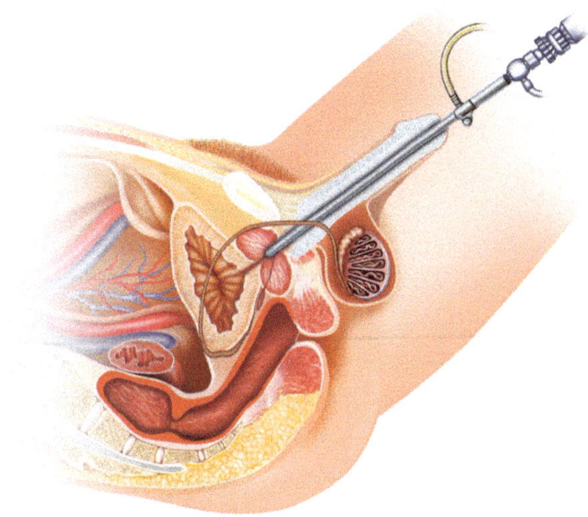

© Alexilusmedical/Shutterstock.com

The process of viewing the urinary bladder is termed a cystoscopy. Cyst/o (bladder) + -scopy (process of viewing). A cystourethroscopy is the visual examination of the bladder and urethra, often with a biopsy of the ureter.

A catheter is a tube that is meant to withdraw or instill a fluid. A straight catheter is removed when urine has been drained, but an indwelling catheter remains in the bladder.

A stent is a tubular device to support hollow structures during a surgical anastomosis, or for holding arteries open after an angioplasty.

The first, a laparoscope, is an instrument to view the abdomen. Lapar/o = abdomen.

The second, a cystoscope, is an instrument to view the urinary bladder. Cyst/o = bladder.

The third, a nephroscope, is an instrument to view the kidney. Nephr/o = kidney.

If stones cause pain or obstruct the flow of urine, they need to be removed. One method is to crush the stones and allow them to flow out of the body along with the urine. The process of crushing stones is termed lithotripsy. Lith/o = stones + -tripsy is the process of crushing.

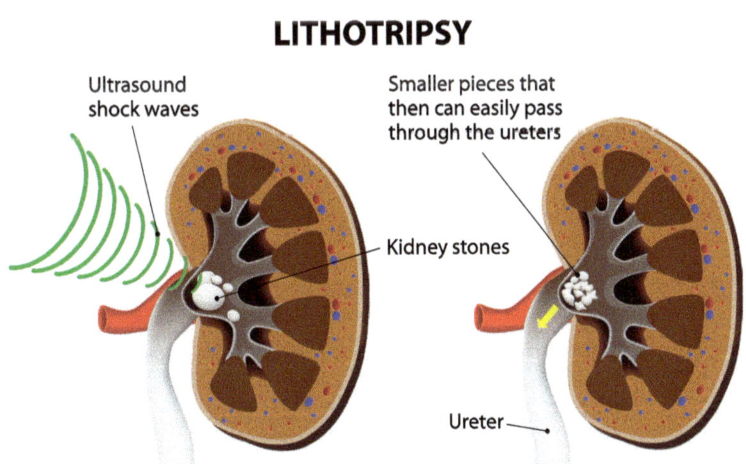

© Designua/Shutterstock.com

Kidney failure can be treated with the surgical transfer of a complete kidney from a donor to a recipient. Notice that the new kidney is placed in the iliac fossa, not in the position of the removed kidney.

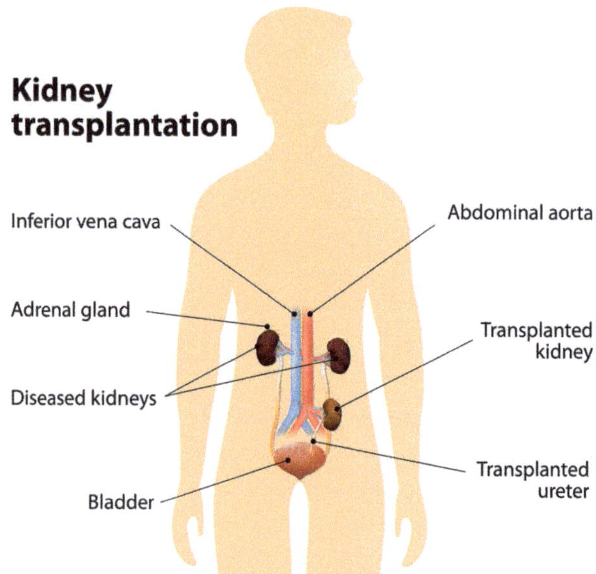

© Designua/Shutterstock.com

CHAPTER 11

Endocrine

The endocrine system is made up of glands, each of which secretes a type of hormone into the bloodstream. The glands of the endocrine system and the hormones they release influence almost every cell, organ, and function of the body. The endocrine glands are the body's main hormone producers. The primary glands of the endocrine system are the pituitary, pineal, thyroid, parathyroid, pancreas, adrenals, ovaries in the female, and testes in the male. The vital function of the endocrine system involves the production and regulation of chemical substances called hormones.

The endocrine (endo- within + -crine = to secrete) glands secrete hormones that act on specific cells called "target cells" at specific sites termed "receptor sites." The hormones and their target cells are similar to a lock and key: both are necessary for the hormones to effect their action.

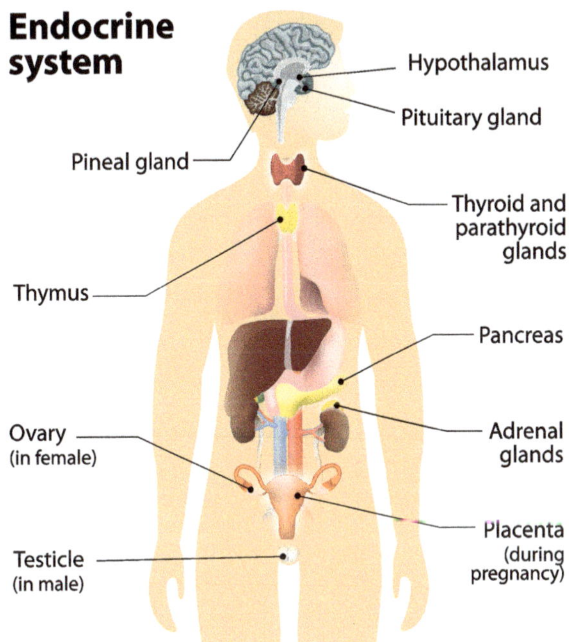

The pituitary gland (also called the hypophysis) is a tiny gland located behind the optic nerve in the cranial cavity.

It is also known as the "master gland" because of its role in controlling other endocrine glands. The name *hypophysis* is the proper anatomic term.

Divided into two lobes, the anterior lobe, called the adenophypophyis, is composed of glandular tissue (aden/o) and secretes hormones in response to stimulation by the hypothalamus. The principal hormones and the target organs on which they act are growth hormone/the bones; adrenocorticotropic hormone/the adrenal cortex; thyroid-stimulating hormone/thyroid; gonadotropic hormone/ovaries and testes; and prolactin/mammary glands.

Be careful! Do not confuse aden/o, which means gland, with adren/o, which means the adrenal gland.

The posterior lobe, the neurohypophysis, is composed of nervous tissue (neur/o) and secretes hormones that it receives from the hypothalamus. The two hormones released by this lobe are antidiuretic hormone (ADH), which acts on the tubules of the kidneys, and oxytocin (OT), which acts on the uterine smooth muscle and the mammary glands.

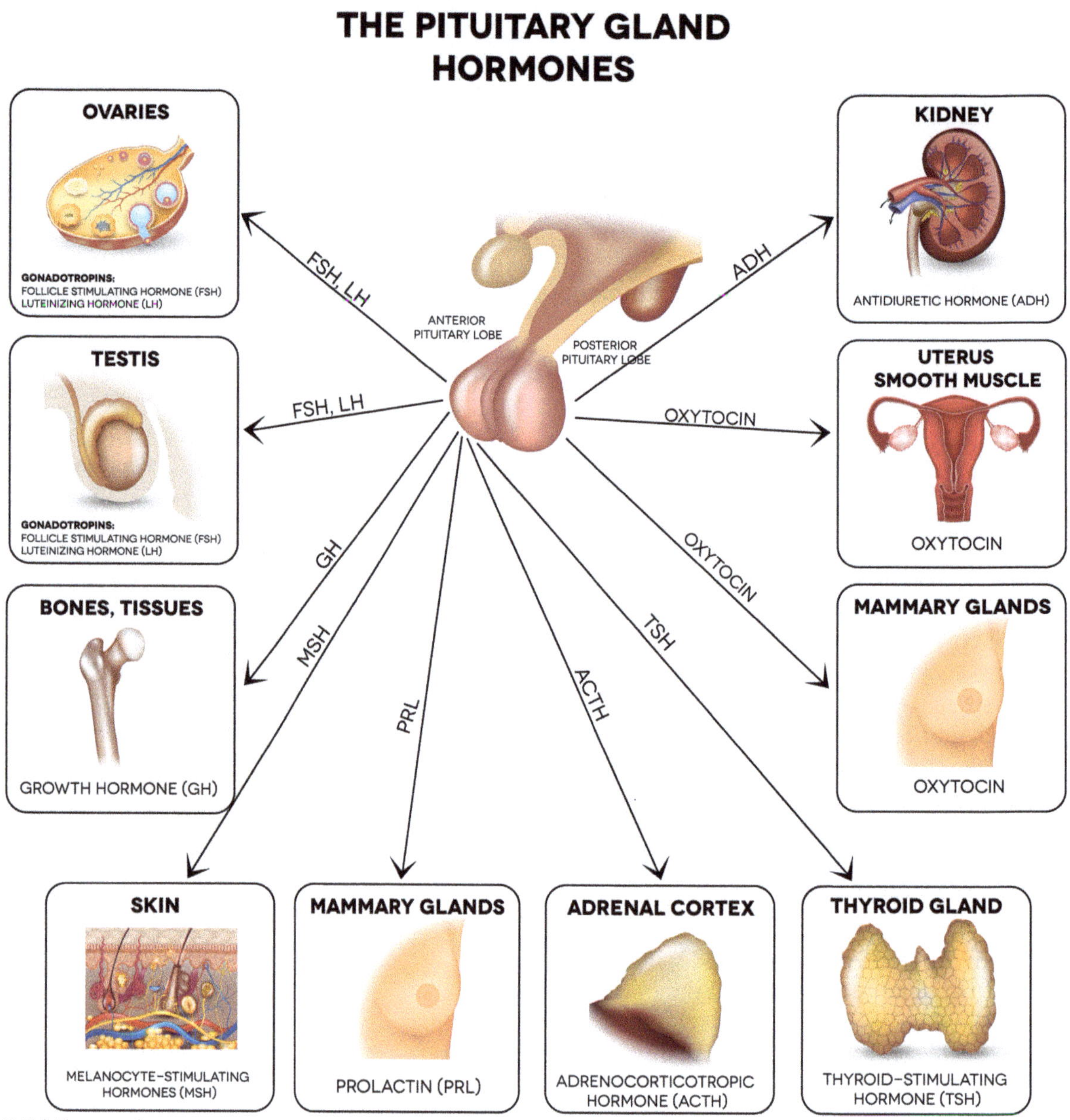

The thyroid gland is a single organ that is located in the anterior part of the neck. It is responsible for metabolism and normal growth and development. It also controls the amount of calcium that is deposited in the bones. The hormones secreted are the following: Calcitonin, which regulates the amount of calcium in the bloodstream; Tetraiodothyronine (thyroxine), which increases cell metabolism; Triiodothyronine, which increases cell metabolism.

The parathyroids are four small glands that are located on the posterior surface of the thyroid gland in the neck. They secrete parathyroid hormone (PTH) in response to a low level of calcium in the blood. If a low level of calcium is detected, PTH increases the level by causing it to be released from the bones. This results in calcium reabsorption by the kidneys and the digestive system. PTH is inhibited by high levels of calcium.

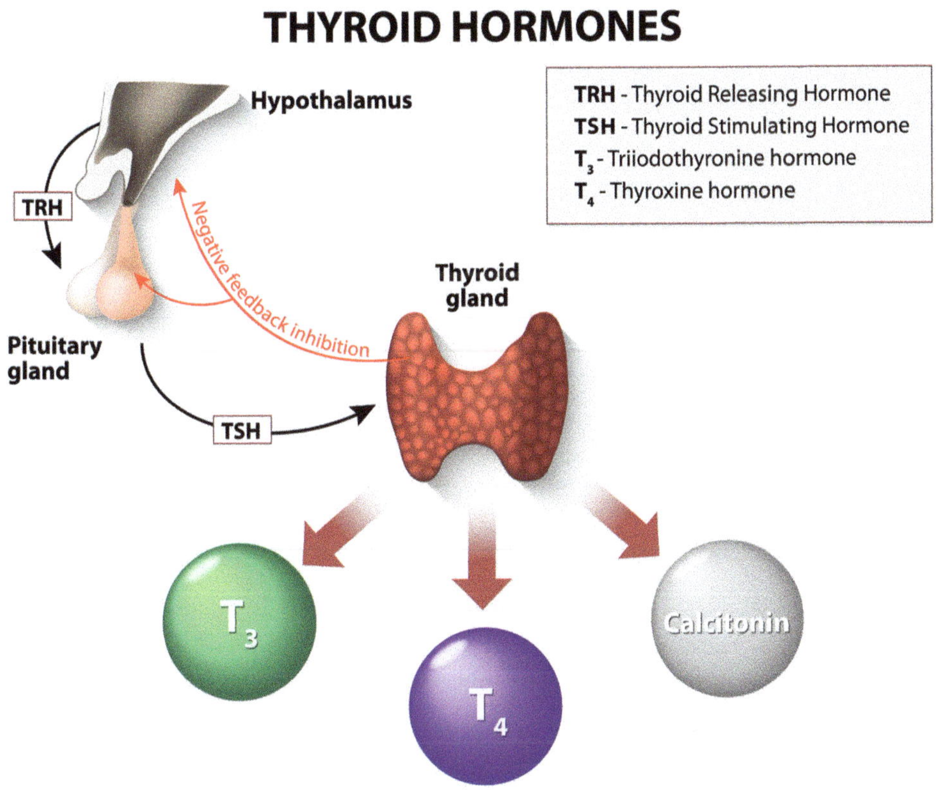

THYROID HORMONES
TRH - Thyroid Releasing Hormone
TSH - Thyroid Stimulating Hormone
T3 - Triiodothyronine hormone
T4 - Thyroxine hormone
Hypothalamus
TRH
Negative feedback inhibition
Thyroid gland
Pituitary gland
TSH
T3
T4
Calcitonin

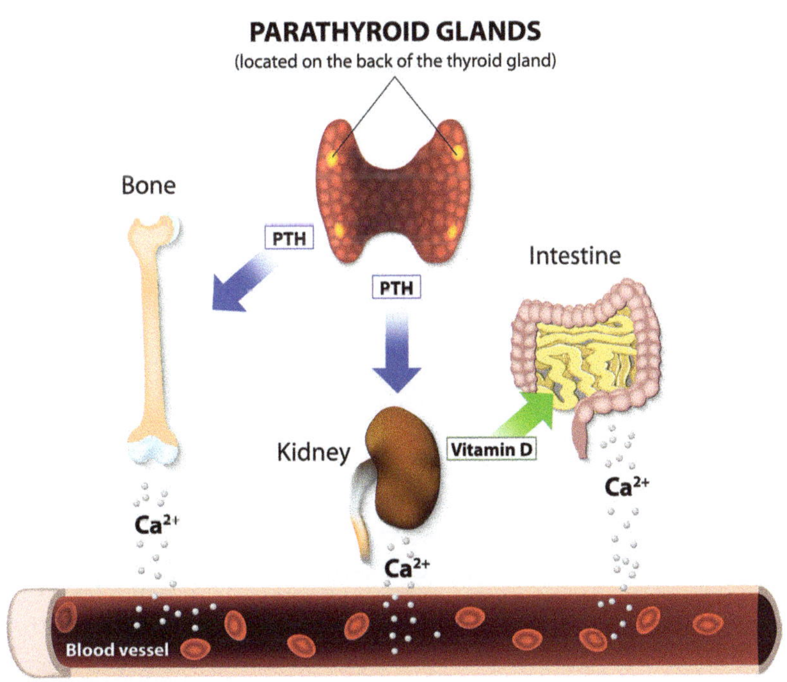

PARATHYROID GLANDS
(located on the back of the thyroid gland)
Bone
PTH
PTH
Intestine
Kidney
Vitamin D
Ca2+
Ca2+
Ca2+
Blood vessel

ADRENAL GLAND
(hormones)

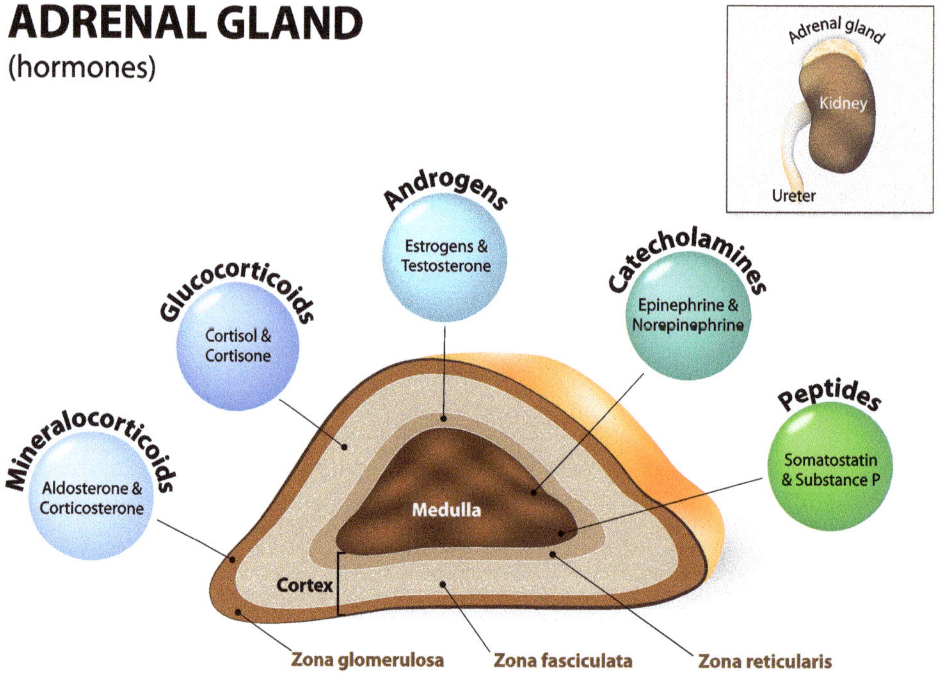

© Designua/Shutterstock.com

The adrenal glands (also called the suprarenals) are paired glands that are located on top of each kidney (ad- = toward + ren/o = kidney). They are composed of an outer part, called the adrenal cortex, and an inner part, called the adrenal medulla.

The adrenal cortex secretes three hormones that are steroids.

The adrenal medulla secretes sympathomimetic hormones that stimulate the fight-or-flight response to stress, similar to the sympathetic nervous system.

The pancreas is located inferior (below) and posterior (behind) to the stomach. It functions as an exocrine gland to release digestive enzymes through a small duct into the small intestines.

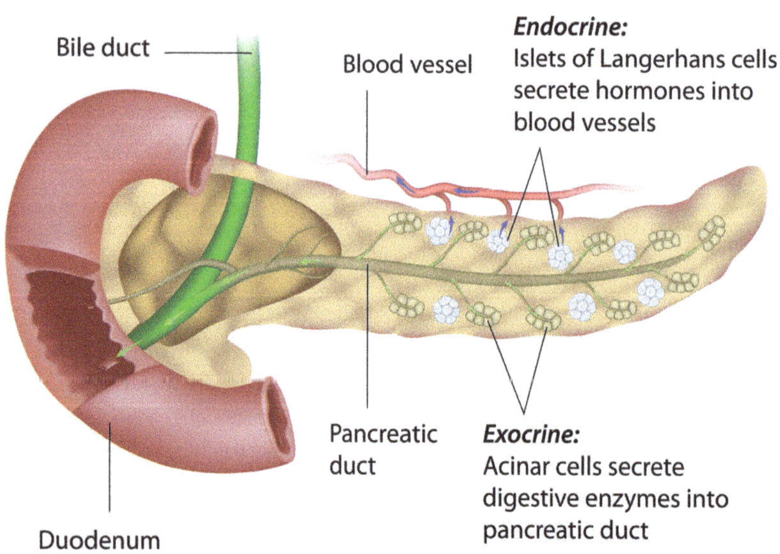

© Alila Medical Media/Shutterstock.com

Its endocrine function, through a variety of cells in the islets of Langerhans, is to regulate the level of glucose in the blood by stimulating the liver.

The alpha cells produce the hormone glucagon, which increases the level of glucose in the blood when levels are low.

The beta cells produce insulin, which decreases the level of glucose in the blood when levels are high.

In the absence of glucose in the cells, proteins and fats are broken down, causing excessive fatty acids and ketones (waste products from the breakdown of fat) in the blood.

The thymus gland is located in the mediastinum above the heart. It releases the hormone thymosin, which is responsible for stimulating key cells in the immune response.

Be careful! Do not confuse thyr/o, which means thyroid, and thym/o, which means thymus.

The ovaries and testes, the female and male gonads, act as endocrine glands to influence reproductive function. The ovaries are located in the pelvic cavity of the female and the testes in the scrotum of the male. These will be discussed in more detail in each chapter on their individual disorders.

The pineal gland is located in the center of the brain, functioning to secrete the hormone melatonin, which is thought to be responsible for inducing sleep.

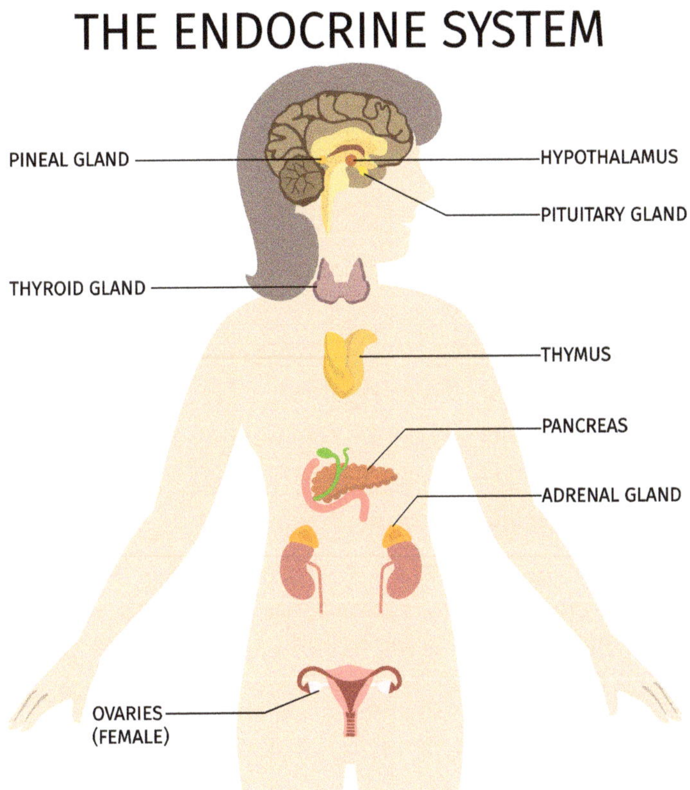

© Creative Mood/Shutterstock.com

Anorexia (an- = without + orex/o = appetite) is a lack of appetite. Don't confuse this with anorexia nervosa, which is an eating disorder.

Exophthalmia (ex- = out + ophthalm/o = eye) is a protrusion of the eyeballs from their orbits.

Goiter is an enlargement of the thyroid gland that is not due to a tumor.

Hirsutism is abnormal hairiness, especially in women. It is also called hypertrichosis (hyper- = excessive + trich/o = hair + -osis = abnormal condition).

Paresthesia (par- = abnormal + esthesi/o = feeling) is an abnormal sensation such as prickling.

Tetany is continuous muscle spasms.

Glucosuria is the presence of sugar (glucose) in the urine. This may indicate diabetes mellitus and is sometimes referred to as glycosuria.

Ketoacidosis is the excessive amount of ketone acids in the bloodstream.

Ketonuria is the presence of ketones in the urine.

Polydipsia is a condition of excessive thirst (dips/o = thirst). Note that *poly-* does not translate well as "many" when the term has to do with thirst, eating, or urination. The meaning "excessive" is suggested in these contexts instead.

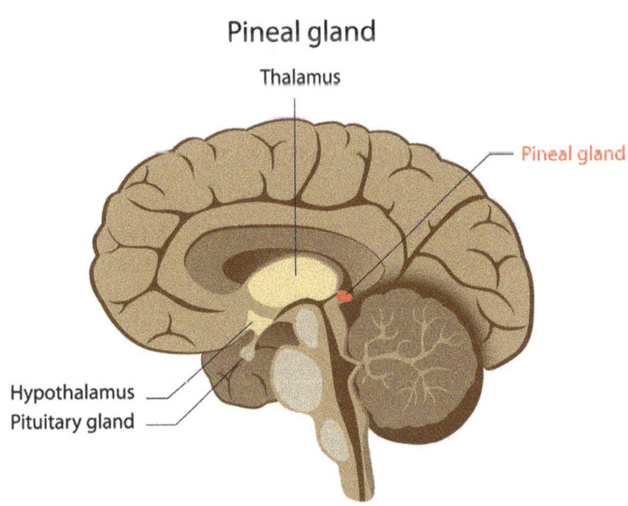

© Alila Medical Media/Shutterstock.com

Polyphagia (phag/o = to eat, swallow) is a condition of excessive appetite.

Polyuria is a condition of excessive urination.

Hypo- in each of the following terms indicates a deficiency, while the prefix hyper- refers to an excessive amount. Note that each of these is also a blood condition (-emia = blood condition).

> Calc/o = calcium
> Glyc/o = glucose
> Kal/i = potassium
> Natr/o = sodium
> Hypocalcemia—Hypercalcemia
> Hypoglycemia—Hyperglycemia
> Hypokalemia—Hyperkalemia
> Hyponatremia—Hypernatremia

Acromegaly (acro- = extremities + -megaly = enlargement) is an enlargement of the extremities (the hands and feet) along with the jaw, nose, and forehead. This is caused by an oversecretion of somatotropin during the adult years. The cause of the oversecretion is usually a benign glandular tumor (adenoma) of the pituitary gland.

Gigantism is a hypersecretion of somatotropin during childhood, leading to an excessive amount of growth.

Growth hormone deficiency (GHD) is an undersecretion of somatotropin due to a dysfunction of the pituitary. This disorder leads to dwarfism. If the deficiency is acquired during adulthood, the patient develops obesity, weakness, and cardiac difficulties.

Hyperparathyroidism is an overproduction of parathyroid hormone. Symptoms include polyuria, hypercalcemia, hypertension, and kidney stones.

Hypoparathyroidism is a deficient amount of parathyroid hormone production resulting in tetany, hypocalcemia, irritability, and muscle cramps.

Addison's disease is an insufficient secretion of adrenal cortisol from the adrenal cortex. Symptoms include gastric complaints, hypotension, and dehydration.

Cushing disease is an excessive secretion of cortisol by the adrenal cortex. Symptoms include obesity, leukocytosis (a slight increase of white blood cells), hirsutism (abnormal hairiness), hyperglycemia, and muscle wasting. The illustration shows the boy before treatment and then four months after treatment was started.

Diabetes mellitus is a group of metabolic disorders characterized by high glucose levels that result from inadequate/ineffective amounts of insulin.

Gestational diabetes (gestation= pregnancy) is insulin resistance by the mother acquired during pregnancy. Although it usually resolves at birth, some of these women are more likely to develop type 2 diabetes later in life.

Hyperinsulinism is an excessive amount of insulin that is seen in some infants at birth. It causes severe hypoglycemia.

Prediabetes is a condition of an elevated blood glucose level, but not high enough for a diagnosis of type 2 diabetes.

Type 1 diabetes is a total lack of insulin production. It results in glycosuria, polydipsia, polyphagia, polyuria, blurred vision, fatigue, and frequent infections. It is currently thought to be an autoimmune disorder. A previous name for type 1 diabetes is insulin-dependent diabetes mellitus (IDDM).

Type 2 diabetes is a deficient amount of insulin production, with symptoms similar to type 1 diabetes. The causes are unknown, but obesity and family history are closely associated with the incidence of the disease. Type 2 diabetes was formerly termed non-insulin-dependent diabetes mellitus (NIDDM).

The A1c (also called glycosylated hemoglobin or HbA1c) is a measure of the average blood glucose during a 3-month time span. It is used to monitor diabetes treatment.

A fasting plasma glucose (formerly called a fasting blood sugar) is a blood test that is done to measure the amount of glucose present in the blood. It measures the body's ability to break down and use glucose. If the measure is between 100 and 125 mg/dL, it indicates a prediabetic state; if it is over 126 mg/dL, it indicates a diagnosis of diabetes.

A glucometer (gluc/o = sugar + -meter = instrument to measure) is an instrument to measure blood sugar.

An oral glucose tolerance test is a blood test to measure the body's response to a concentrated glucose solution. It is used to diagnose diabetes mellitus.

A urine glucose test is used to screen for or to monitor diabetes mellitus. A urine specimen is examined for the presence of glucose.

If a urine specimen is positive for urine ketones, their presence may indicate diabetes mellitus or hyperthyroidism.

Hormone tests examine the quantity of various hormones in the blood to diagnose or monitor a disease. Examples are antidiuretic hormone, cortisol, growth hormone, or parathyroid hormone.

Radioimmunoassay studies are nuclear medicine tests to tag and detect hormones in the blood through the use of radionuclides.

Thyroid function tests are blood tests done to assess triiodothyronine, tetraiodothyronine (thyroxine), and calcitonin. They may be used to assess abnormalities of thyroid function.

Total calcium is a measure of the amount of calcium in the blood. Results may be used to assess parathyroid function, calcium metabolism, or cancerous conditions.

Urinalysis is a physical, chemical, and microscopic examination of the urine. Urine glucose and urine ketones are two substances that may be present to indicate difficulties with pancreatic function.

Computed tomography may be used to test for bone density in hypoparathyroidism or for measuring the size of the adrenal glands in Addison's disease.

Magnetic resonance imaging may be used to examine changes in the size of soft tissue; for example, the pituitary, pancreas, or hypothalamus.

Radioactive iodine (RAI) uptake scans are done to test thyroid function by measuring the gland's ability to concentrate and retain iodine. It is useful in diagnosing hyperthyroidism.

Radiography (x-rays) is used to examine suspected changes that affect the density or thickness of bone. It may also be used to reveal underlying causes of an endocrine disorder.

Sonography is used to visualize the pancreas and to guide biopsies of the thyroid gland when determining if cysts are solid or fluid filled.

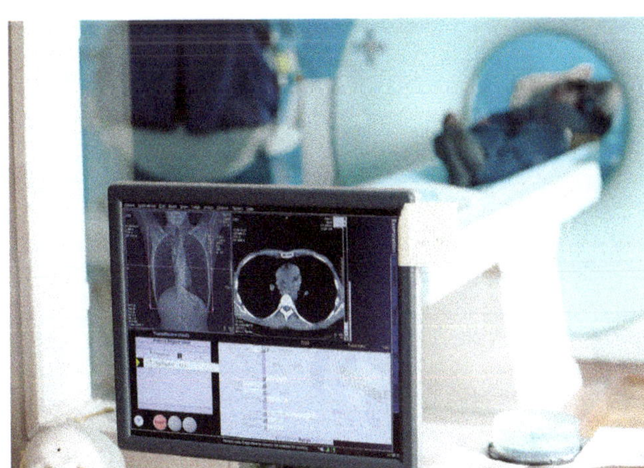

CHAPTER 12

Male Reproductive System

The male reproductive system consists of the testes, epididymis, vas deferens, and urethra. The supporting structures and accessory sex organs are the scrotum and penis. The vital function of the male reproductive system is to provide sperm cells necessary to fertilize the ovum.

The function of the male reproductive system is to reproduce! The male provides half of the genetic information.

Andr/o = male + -logy = study of. Andrology is the study of males, usually in regard to fertility issues.

Ur/o = urinary system + -logy = study of.

Urology is the study of the urinary system; many of men's health issues are treated by a urologist.

Genitalia is a term that means reproductive organs. It is made up of two types of tissue: parenchymal and stromal.

Remember that parenchymal tissue does the work of the system. In this case, the parenchymal tissue of the male reproductive system is the male gonad, the testicle, which produces the male gamete, the spermatozoa. The testes produce the sperm through the process of spermatogenesis (spermat/o = sperm + -genesis = production), which is triggered by the male hormone, testosterone (test/o = testis + ster/o = steroid + -one = hormone). Testosterone is produced in the interstitial cells of the testicles beginning in puberty.

The stromal tissue is supportive; it includes the numerous glands that provide fluid for the spermatozoa, the vessels that provide a blood supply, the ducts that carry sperm out of the body, and the nerves that provide the innervation to the structures involved.

Let's start with the sac that holds the testes, called the scrotum. Next is the testis (pl. testes), the organ that is referred to as the male gonad. Again, this is the organ that produces the male gametes, the spermatozoa. Notice that it is covered by a membrane called the tunica vaginalis. Vaginalis here refers to a "sheath"–NOT to a female reproductive structure, but the term does

Male Reproductive System

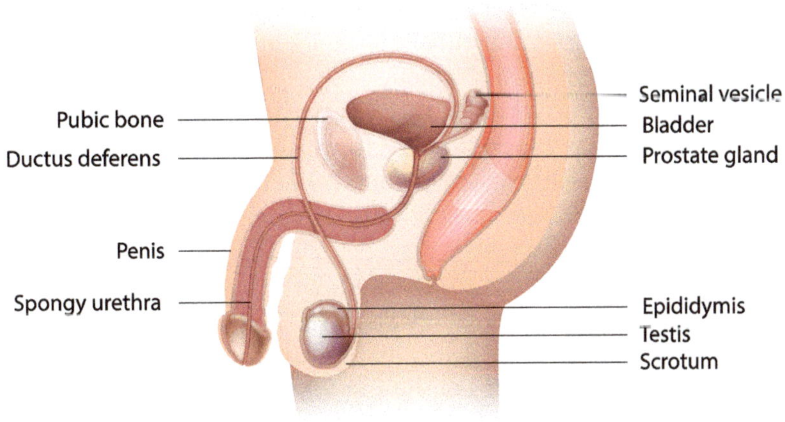

© BlueRingMedia/Shutterstock.com

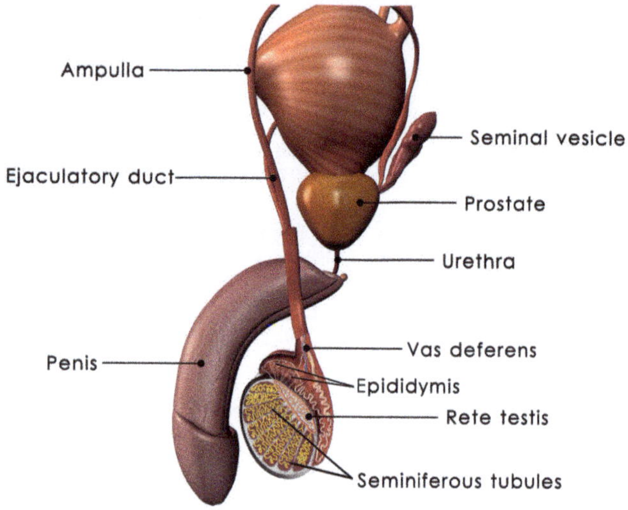

share the same word origin. You can see the epididymis and the vas deferens. Remember that these are paired organs. You are seeing only one here.

The vas deferens conducts the sperm around the bladder to the area of the seminal vesicles where it picks up fluid for nourishment, then on to the urethra. The urethra continues through the penis and is surrounded by columns of tissue called the corpus cavernosa and the corpus spongiosum. These columns fill with blood during sexual excitement and are responsible for an erection of the penis. The end of the penis is termed the glans penis (no "d" in glans) and the skin surrounding it is called the prepuce (commonly called the foreskin).

These are the sites of sperm production.

At the top of the testicle is the epididymis. This is the area in which the sperm are stored until they are released through ejaculation.

The vas deferens (also called the ductus deferens) is the vessel that conducts sperm out of each testicle. The spermatic cord is a sheath that includes the vas deferens along with nerves and blood vessels.

The sperm start in the testes, travel to the vas deferens, pass through the seminal vesicle, and proceed to the ejaculatory duct. This duct opens during ejaculation, closing off the passage of urine into the urethra. The sperm then continues out through the urethra, exiting through the urinary meatus.

Gonad/o is the combining form for gonad, the general term for a sex organ. In the male it's the testis or testicle; in the female it is the ovary.

The combining forms for the testicles are test/o, testicul/o, orchid/o, orch/o, and orchi/o.

Seminiferous in seminiferous tubules is built from the combining form for semen, semin/i, and the suffix –ferous meaning to bear or to carry.

The sex cells are the gametes. In the male, they are called spermatozoa (singular: spermatozoon). The production of sperm is spermatogenesis. Spermat/o = sperm + -genesis = production.

Semen is the combination of sperm and the fluid in which it is bathed. As mentioned, semin/i is the combining form for semen.

The combining form for the sac that holds the testicles outside of the body is scrot/o.

Epididym/o is the combining form for the vessels that store the sperm, and vas/o and duct/o are used to represent the vas (or ductus) deferens.

The spermatic cord does not have a combining form, but we shall see that it can involve a specific, serious condition.

The combining form for the seminal vesicles is vesicul/o. The seminal vesicles, bulbourethral glands (also called Cowper's glands), and the prostate gland (combining form prostat/o) provide fluid for the nutrition and motility (movement) of the sperm.

Pen/i and phall/o are combining forms for the penis. You will probably rarely see them used, except in their adjectival form as penile and phallic.

The combining form for the glans penis (balan/o) is one of the word parts most commonly forgotten by the end of the term. Can you think of a way to remember this one?

The final combining form for stromal tissue is preputi/o for the foreskin. Again, you will probably see this in its adjectival form as preputial.

The ejaculatory duct does not have its own combining form.

Prostate is the gland—not to be confused with prostrate, a word that means someone is lying face down!

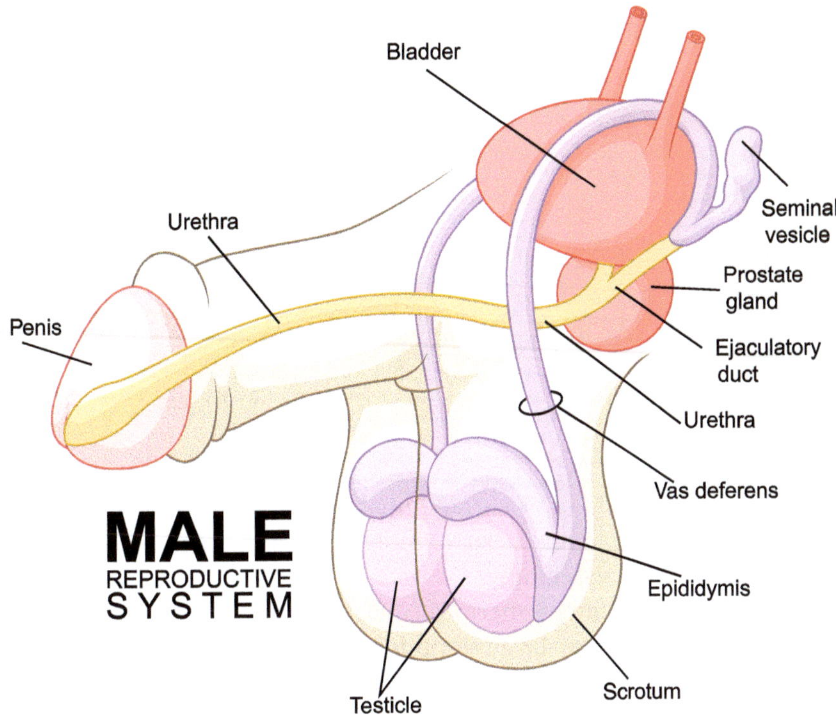

© rendix_alextian/Shutterstock.com

Vesic/o means urinary bladder and vesicul/o means vesicle.

The normal method of reproduction is through sexual intercourse. Two other terms that are synonyms are coitus and copulation.

An- (no, not, without) + orchid/o (testicle) + -ism (condition). A condition of no testicle. It may be stated as unilateral (pertaining to one side) or bilateral (pertaining to two sides). The fertility of an individual is not compromised if one testicle remains.

Chordee (chord/o = cord) is a congenital defect resulting in a downward curvature of the penis due to a fibrous band (cord) of tissue along the corpus spongiosum.

Crypt- (hidden) + orchid/o (testicle) + -ism (condition). A condition of a "hidden" or undescended testicle.

Epispadias is an abnormal condition of the opening of the urethra on the dorsum of the penis (epi- meaning above or on top of).

A synonym is hyperspadias, Hyper- (above) + -spadias (condition of a rent or tear).

Hypo- (under) + -spadias (condition of a rent or tear). This is an abnormal condition of the opening of the urethra on the underside (ventral side) of the penis.

Phimosis literally means "to muzzle." This is a condition, usually congenital, of a tightening of the foreskin over the glans penis. This tightening restricts the flow of

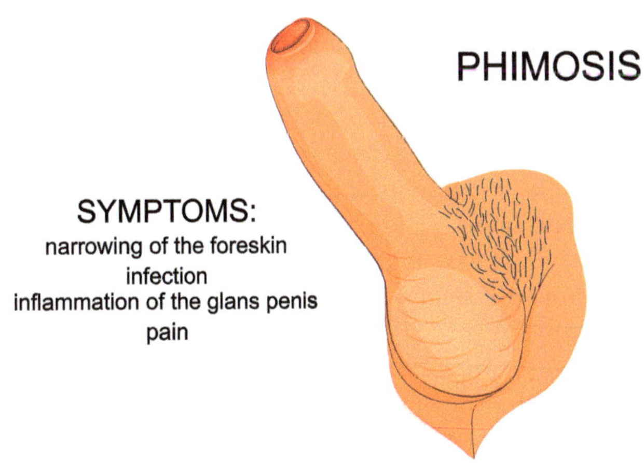

© Artemida-psy/Shutterstock.com

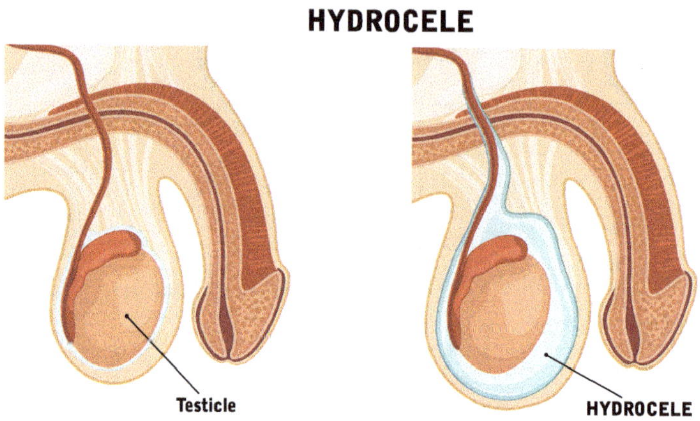

© logika600/Shutterstock.com

urine and semen from the urinary meatus. The correction is a circumcision (circum- = around, -cision = processing of cutting).

A- (no, not, without) + sperm/o (spermatozoa) + -ia (condition). Aspermia is a condition of no sperm AND no semen being emitted during ejaculation. This one is a little tricky, because there is no reference to semen in the term itself.

A- (no, not, without) + zo/o (animal) + sperm/o (spermatozoa) + -ia (condition). Azoospermia is a condition of no living sperm (animal life!) in the semen. This is a desired condition in individuals who have had a vasectomy.

Olig/o (scanty, few) + sperm/o (spermatozoa) + -ia (condition). Oligospermia is a condition of scanty sperm. This may be a reason for a couple's infertility.

A hydrocele is a protrusion in the scrotum due to an accumulation of fluid in the tunica vaginalis. Hydr/o (fluid, water) + -cele (herniation, protrusion).

A varicocele is an abnormal dilation of the veins of the spermatic cord. Varic/o [varices (swollen, twisted veins)] + -cele (herniation, protrusion).

Notice that each of these terms ends in the suffix *–itis*, meaning inflammation.

Epididymitis is an inflammation of the epididymis (epididym/o = epididymis), the area in which sperm are stored above the testes.

Orchitis is an inflammation of the testes (orch/o = testis) and may or may not be associated with the mumps virus. A synonym is testitis.

Prostatitis is an inflammation of the prostate gland (prostat/o = prostate).

Vesiculitis is an inflammation of the seminal vesicles (vesicul/o = seminal vesicle).

Balanitis is an inflammation of the glans penis (balan/o = glans penis).

Testicular torsion is the twisting of a testicle on its spermatic cord, usually because of trauma.

Gynecomastia is female-like breast tissue in a male.

Erectile dysfunction is the inability to achieve or sustain a penile erection.

Priapism is an abnormally prolonged erection.

BPH is benign prostatic hyperplasia (also called benign prostatic hypertrophy). Hyper- = excessive + -plasia = condition of formation, development. An overgrowth of prostatic tissue, although benign and characteristically not prone to spread, can cause the urethra to be narrowed or closed. It is a common disorder in men older than 50 years of age.

Gon/o = seed + -rrhea = flow, discharge. Gonorrhea is a term that has changed its meaning over time. A sexually transmitted disease, gonorrhea is marked by a mucopurulent (mucous and pus filled) discharge. Initially, it was thought that this discharge was of semen containing sperm. Hence the use of gon/o meaning seed. Gonorrhea is caused by the gram-negative diplococcus *Neisseria gonorrhoeae* bacteria, which can infect the urethra, prostate, rectum, and pharynx. In women, it can involve the cervix and fallopian tubes and may be asymptomatic (*a-* no, not, without), meaning that it has no symptoms.

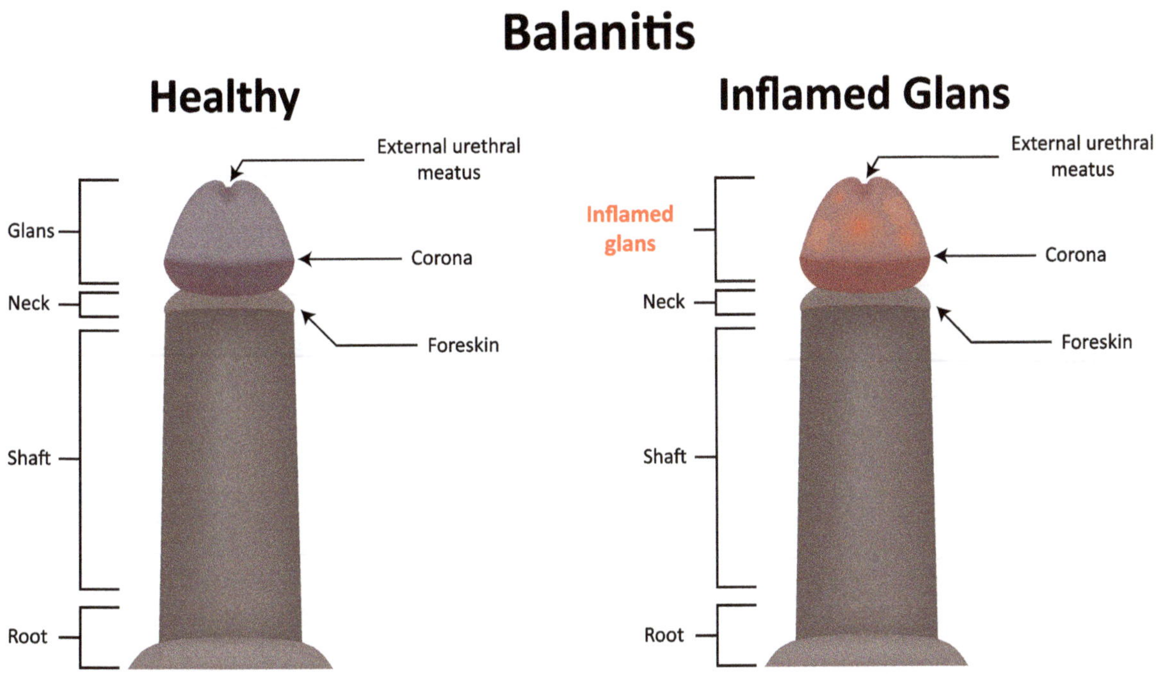

Syphilis is a multistage sexually transmitted disease caused by a spirochete, *Treponema pallidum*. The first sign of this disease may be a painless red pustule, called a chancre, that usually appears on the genitals.

HSV-2 is a form of the herpesvirus that is spread through sexual contact. It causes painful vesicular (blister-like) eruptions.

HPV is a virus that causes warts of the hands, feet, and mucous membranes. Genital warts are referred to as condyloma (pl. condylomata).

NGU is an inflammation of the urethra (urethr/o = urethra + -itis = inflammation); it is named by what it is NOT caused by (gonorrhea). The pathogens that do cause it are *Chlamydia trachomatis*, *Mycoplasma genitalium*, and *Ureaplasma urealyticum*.

Each of these can be used to detect an enlargement of the prostate gland.

A DRE is a digital rectal examination, in which a gloved finger is inserted into the rectum to palpate the prostate.

A PSA is a blood test to test the increased levels of an antigen that may indicate prostate cancer. PSA stands for prostate-specific antigen.

Transrectal sonography is the use of high-frequency sound waves to image the prostate. Trans = through, across + rect/o = rectum + -al = pertaining to. The transducer (the unit that is inserted into the rectum) makes its images through the rectum.

Vas/o (vas deferens or ductus deferens) + -ectomy (removal). A vasectomy is the cutting, tying, and burning shut of the ends of both vas deferens.

Vas/o (vas deferens) + vas/o (vas deferens) + -stomy (new opening). A vasovasostomy is a reversal of a vasectomy, in which a "new" opening is made between previously cut, tied, and burned shut ends of the vas deferens.

Prostat/o (prostate gland) + -ectomy (removal). A prostatectomy is a removal of the prostate gland.

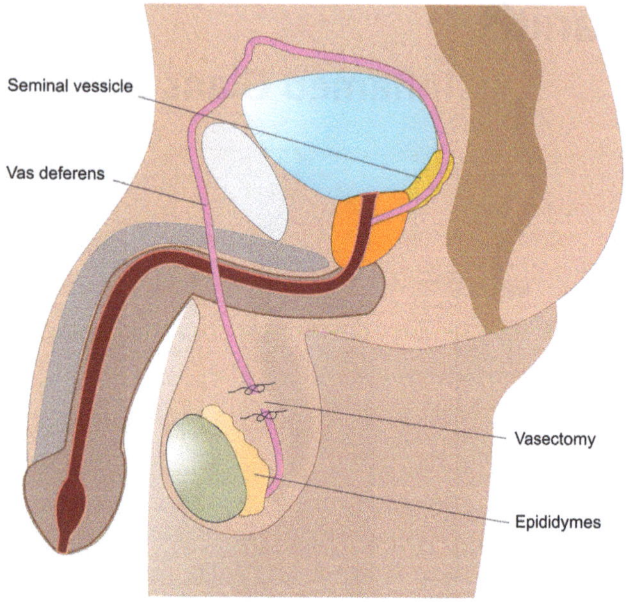

© ellepigrafica/Shutterstock.com

TUIP stands for transurethral incision of the prostate gland. Trans- = through + urethr/ = urethra + -al = pertaining to. This procedure involves a series of incisions that are made through the urethra into the prostate gland in order to reduce its pressure on the urethra. It is NOT removed in this procedure.

TURP stands for transurethral resection of the prostate. Again, transurethral means through the prostate, but here the prostate is removed (resection). This is an extremely common procedure for benign prostatic hyperplasia (BPH).

Ablation is a general term meaning removal of tissue by a variety of means: surgical, chemical destruction, electrocautery, radiofrequency energy, and through the use of a cryo (extreme cold) probe.

Antibiotics are used to treat bacterial infections (such as syphilis). Examples are penicillin G, tetracycline, and doxycycline.

Antifungals are used to treat fungi (e.g., tinea cruris: jock itch). Butenafine (Lotrimin) and terbinafine (Lamisil) are examples.

Antivirals are used to treat viruses. An example that has gotten a lot of media attention is Zovirax (acyclovir) to treat genital herpes.

Antiimpotence agents are used to alleviate erectile dysfunction. Sildenafil (Viagra), tadalafil (Cialis), and vardenafil (Levitra) are the oral agents currently available. Alprostadil (Caverject) is injected directly into the corpus cavernosum of the penis.

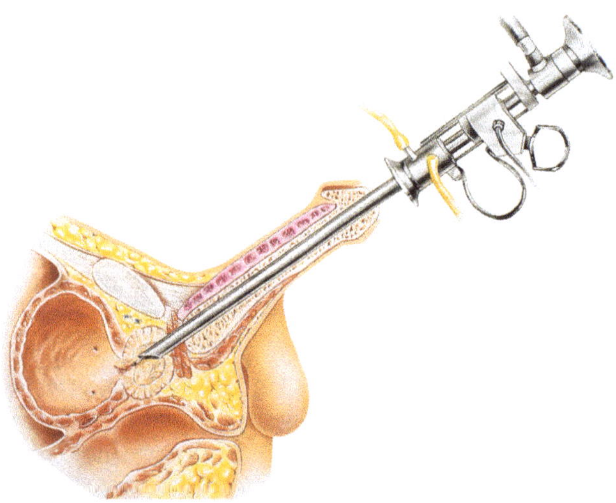

© Medical Art Inc/Shutterstock.com

Alpha-adrenergic inhibitors target alpha-1-adrenergic receptors to relax smooth muscle in the prostate to improve urinary flow. Examples include tamsulosin (Flomax) and terazosin (Hytrin).

Androgen hormone inhibitors block the conversion of testosterone to the more potent hormone 5-alpha-dihydrotestosterone (DHT) to suppress growth of and even shrink the enlarged prostate. Examples include finasteride (Proscar) and dutasteride (Avodart).

CHAPTER 13

Female Reproductive System

The female reproductive system consists of left and right ovaries, which are the primary sex organs of female. The accessory sex organs are the following: two fallopian tubes, the uterus, the vagina, the vulva, and two breasts. The vital function of the female reproductive system is to perpetuate the species through sexual reproduction.

Obstetricians treat women during pregnancy and childbirth.

Gynecologists are medical doctors who monitor health and treat diseases of the female reproductive system.

Midwives assist women through labor and delivery.

Doulas care for a pregnant woman through labor and delivery. They also provide care for the mother and child.

The role of the female reproductive system is to keep her genetic material in the world's gene pool.

The female gamete, the ovum, provides 23 pairs of chromosomes to be combined with the male gamete, the spermatozoon, and its 23 pairs of chromosomes to create a new life.

Once the gamete is fertilized, the female reproductive system functions to nurture the fertilized ovum to delivery.

The ovum is the female gamete (remember that the spermatozoon is the male gamete).

The release of an ovum is termed ovulation.

The ovaries are the female gonads, the small, almond-shaped, paired organs located on either side of the uterus in the pelvic cavity, that produce the ova.

Approximately every 28 days, in response to hormonal stimulation, the ovaries alternate in releasing an ovum. The egg matures in a tiny secretory sac within the ovary called a follicle. If the egg is not fertilized, the lining of the uterus that has been formed to receive the fertilized egg is shed in a process termed menstruation.

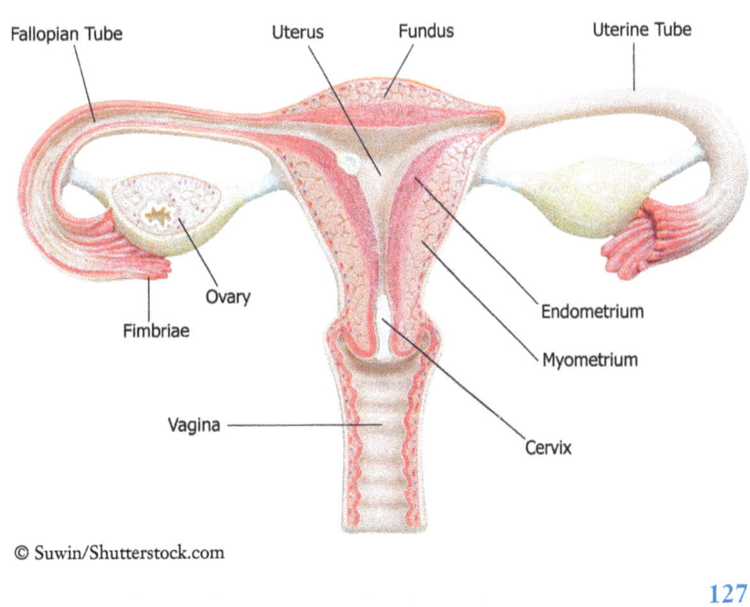

© Suwin/Shutterstock.com

Menarche is the term for the first menstrual period, which

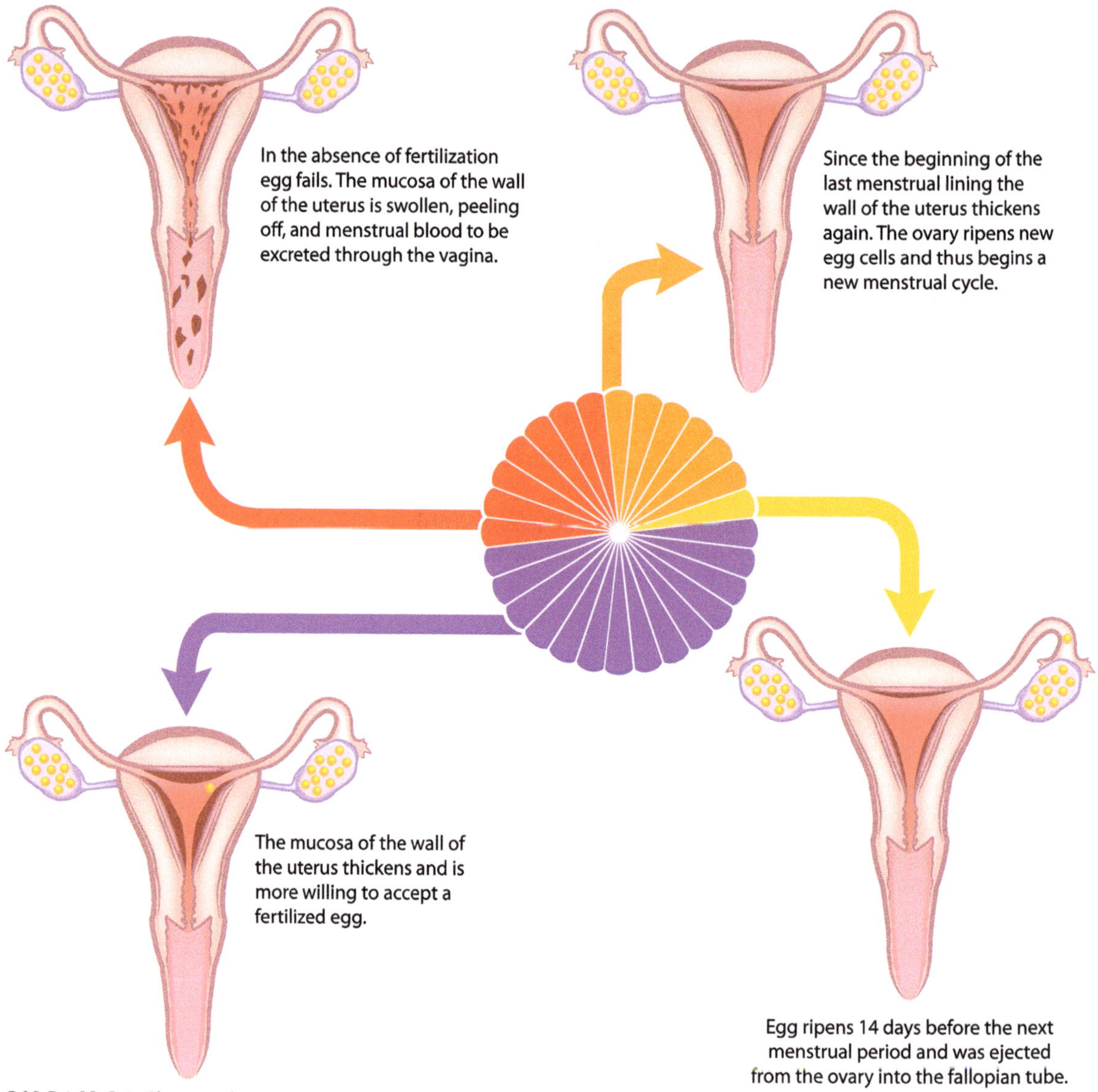

signals the beginning of a woman's fertility. Menopause refers to the ending of menstruation and the end of a woman's fertile period.

The female gonads, the ovaries, are influenced by the secretion of two hormones from the pituitary gland.

Follicle-stimulating hormone (FSH) causes the ovarian follicles to begin to mature and secrete estrogen. The presence of estrogen causes the pituitary to secrete luteinizing hormone, which stimulates the follicle to mature and release its ovum in a process called ovulation.

Luteinizing hormone is also instrumental in the development of the corpus luteum, a structure that develops in the follicles after they rupture, and serves to secrete estrogen and progesterone. These hormones are responsible for female secondary sex characteristics (breast development) and the cyclical maintenance of the uterus for pregnancy.

The internal anatomy continues with the fallopian tubes, two thin tubes about 10–12 cm long, that join the ovaries to the uterus. Other names for the fallopian tubes are the oviducts or uterine tubes. Note that the word parts for the fallopian tubes are salping/o and –salpinx.

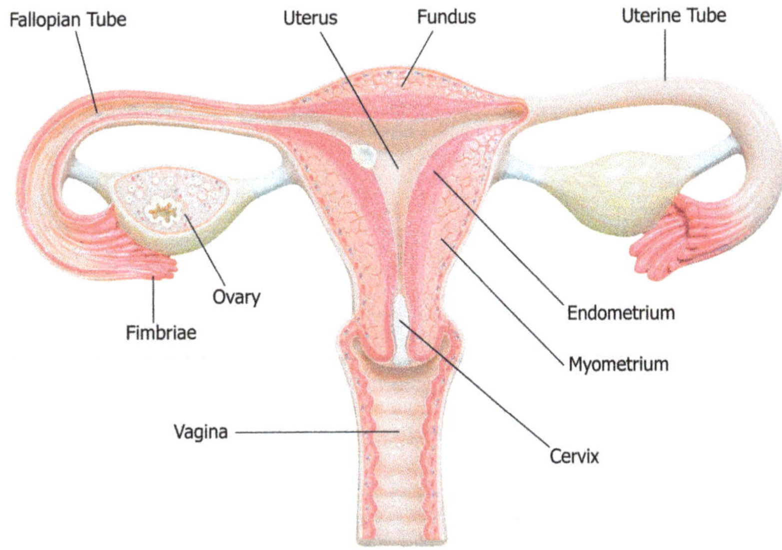

The uterus, or womb, is a pear-shaped organ that serves to nurture the developing embryo/fetus. It is composed of three layers: the inner lining called the endometrium, the muscle layer called the myometrium, and the outer layer called the perimetrium. Note that each of their combining forms is built from a combining form for uterus (metri/o) plus a prefix (endo-, peri-) or another combining form (my/o). Be careful not to confuse –metry (which means the process of measuring) with metr/o (which is the combining form for the uterus).

The cervix is the lowered narrow part of the uterus, often referred to as the neck of the uterus. Be careful to remember that cervic/o has two meanings—neck and cervix.

The rectouterine pouch is the space in the pelvic cavity between the uterus and the rectum. It is also referred to as Douglas' cul-de-sac.

Finally, the vagina is a muscular, tube-like structure at the entrance/exit to the internal female genitalia.

Note that the combining forms for the vagina and the rectouterine pouch look somewhat similar (colp/o and culd/o).

The external genitalia of the female is called the vulva.

It is composed of the vaginal opening (or orifice), the membrane that covers the opening (the hymen), and the two folds of skin that surround the opening: the labia minora (small "lips") and labia majora (large "lips").

The clitoris is the sensitive erectile tissue that is anterior to the urethra.

The Bartholin glands are paired mucous glands that secrete a lubricant.

The mons pubis is the fatty cushion of tissue over the pubic bone.

The perineum is the area between the opening of the vaginal orifice and the anus.

The breasts (mammary glands) function to secrete milk. The breast tissue is composed of glandular milk-producing fatty and fibrous tissue. The nipple of the breast is called the mammary papilla and the darker area around the nipple is called the areola.

Note the significance of the breast quadrants in regard to breast cancer (a method of naming the location of the tumor).

Terms used to refer to sexual intercourse are coitus and copulation.

The fertilization of the ovum by a spermatozoon is termed conception.

The word parts for pregnancy (gestation) are gravid/o, -gravida, and -cyesis.

Once fertilized, the zygote, a fertilized egg, continues to divide and travel through the fallopian tubes to the uterus. This takes approximately 2 weeks.

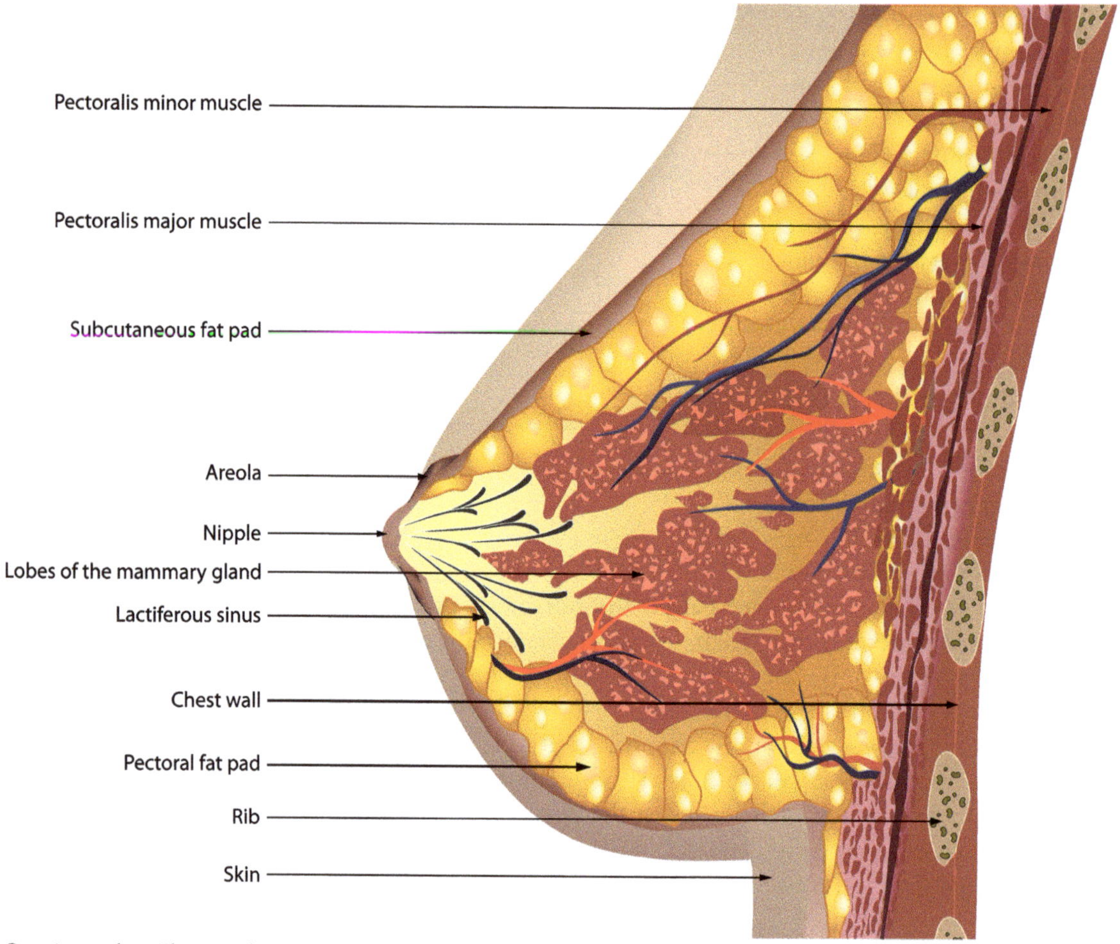

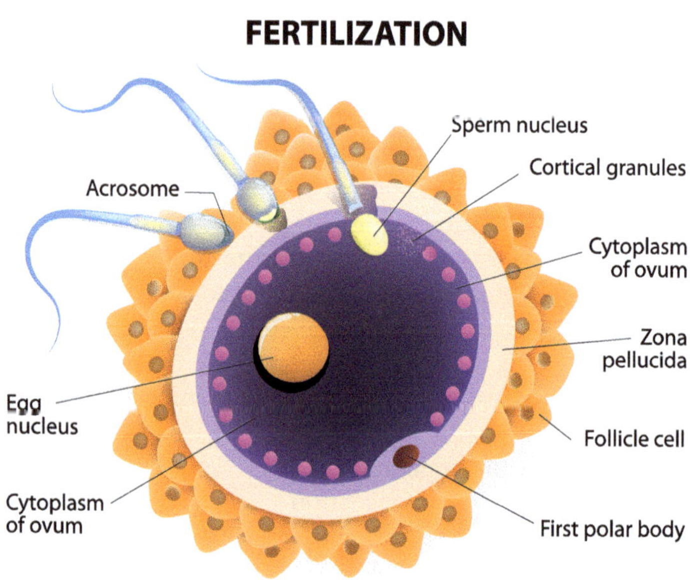

From the third to the eighth week of life, it is called an embryo, and from the ninth week until delivery at approximately 38 weeks, the term given is a fetus.

Human chorionic gonadotropin (hCG) is secreted by the zygote and serves the function of preventing the corpus luteum from deteriorating. This allows the continued production of estrogen and progesterone to support the pregnancy and prevent menstruation.

Extraembryonic structures are those that are outside (extra-) of the embryo.

The amnion is the inner sac or membrane that surrounds the embryo; it contains amniotic fluid that helps to cushion, protect, and allow the embryo room for movement.

The chorion is the outer membrane surrounding the embryo that is continuous with the placenta, the highly vascular structure that acts as a physical communication between the mother and the embryo.

The umbilical cord is the tissue that connects the embryo to the placenta (and hence to the mother). When this cord is cut, the baby is dependent on his or her own body for all physiologic processes. The remaining "scar" is the umbilicus or navel.

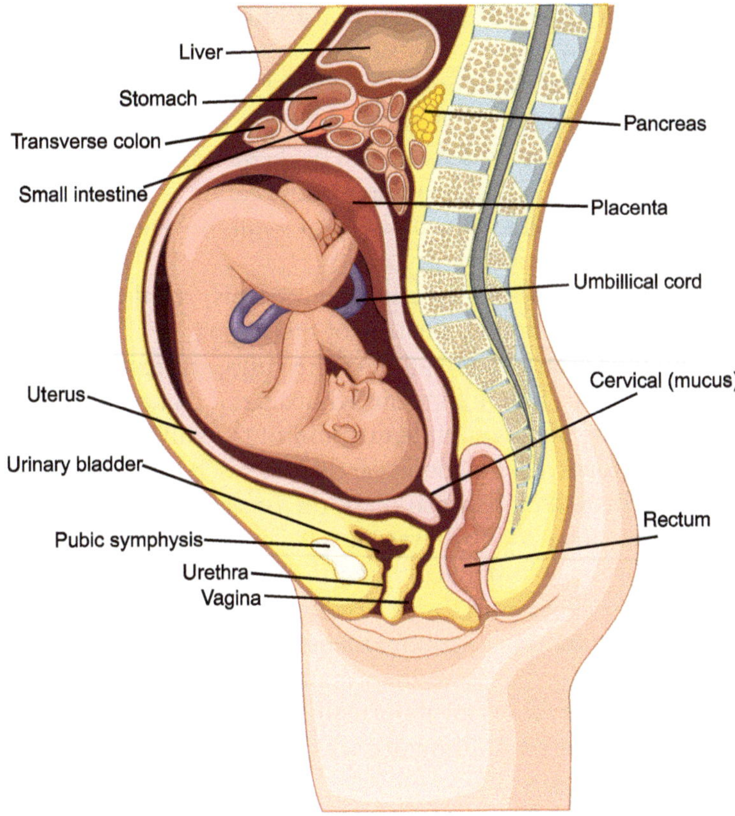

Primigravida means first pregnancy (primi- = first + -gravida = pregnancy).

Multigravida means more than one pregnancy (multi- = many, although many is more than one in this term).

Nulligravida means no pregnancies (nulli- =none).

Parturition (-para, part/o, -partum)

<37 weeks – premature infant

<2500 g – low-birth-weight infant

Parturition is the delivery of an infant. Note the combining forms.

Primipara means first delivery (primi- = first).

Multipara means more than one delivery (multi- = many, although in this term, simple means more than one).

Nullipara is no deliveries (nulli- = none).

Antenatal (ante- before, in front of + nat/o = birth + -al = pertaining to) means pertaining to before birth. Prenatal (pre- = before) means the same thing.

Postnatal (post- = after) means pertaining to after birth.

Antepartum (part/o = parturition, delivery) means before delivery.

Postpartum means after delivery.

Anovulation is the failure of the ovary to release an ovum.

Discuss the possible causes of anovulation.

Oophoritis (oophor/o = ovary) is an inflammation of an ovary.

Polycystic ovary syndrome (PCOS) (poly- = many + cyst/o = sac) is the bilateral presence of numerous cysts caused by a hormonal abnormality leading to the secretion of androgens. PCOS can cause acne, facial hair, and infertility.

Adhesions of the fallopian tubes are scar tissue that bind the inner surfaces of the tubes together. This may be a result of pelvic inflammatory disease (PID), which, as a result of inflammation, may cause the tubes to heal closed, causing infertility.

Hematosalpinx is a condition of blood in the fallopian tubes (hemat/o = blood + -salpinx = fallopian tube).

Hydrosalpinx is a condition of fluid in the fallopian tubes (hydr/o = fluid).

Pyosalpinx is a condition of pus in the fallopian tubes (py/o = pus).

Salpingitis is an inflammation of the fallopian tubes.

Cervicitis is an inflammation of the cervix.

Leukorrhea is a whitish discharge (leuk/o = white + -rrhea = flow, discharge), usually as a result of a cervical inflammation.

Vaginal prolapse (also called colpoptosis) is a downward displacement of the vagina.

Vaginitis is an inflammation of the vagina.

Vulvitis is an inflammation of the vulva, the external female genitalia.

Vulvodynia is an idiopathic syndrome of complaints of pain (-dynia) of the vulva.

Vulvovaginitis is an inflammation of the vulva and the vagina.

Galactorrhea is an abnormal flow or discharge of milk (galact/o = milk) from the breast.

Mastitis is an inflammation of the breast.

Mastoptosis is a downward displacement of the breasts.

Thelitis is an inflammation of the nipple. A synonym is acromastitis.

Amenorrhea is the absence of menstruation.

Dysmenorrhea is a painful menstrual flow.

Oligomenorrhea is an abnormally light or infrequent menstrual flow.

Polymenorrhea is an abnormally frequent menstrual flow.

Agalactia is a condition of a mother's inability to produce milk (a- = without, galact/o = milk + -ia = condition).

Cephalopelvic disproportion is a condition in which the infant's head (cephal/o) is larger than the pelvic outlet through which it must pass. It is one of the indications for a Cesarean section.

Eclampsia is an extreme form of hypertension secondary to pregnancy. Patients are at risk for coma, convulsions, and death.

Preeclampsia is an abnormal condition of pregnancy with an unknown cause. It is marked by hypertension (high blood pressure), edema (swelling), and proteinuria (protein in the urine). Another name for preeclampsia is toxemia of pregnancy.

A miscarriage or abortion is the termination of a pregnancy before the fetus is viable. A spontaneous abortion is a miscarriage; if the miscarriage is induced, it is termed as a therapeutic abortion.

An ectopic pregnancy is an implantation of the embryo in any location other than the uterus. Ec- = out + top/o= place, hence it is a pregnancy out of its normal place. Because 95% of ectopic pregnancies occur in the fallopian tubes, these are also called tubal pregnancies.

Abruptio placentae is the premature separation of the placenta from the uterine wall. This separation can cause a severe hemorrhage that can threaten the lives of the mother and the infant. A synonym is ablatio placentae.

Placenta previa is a malpositioned placenta that covers the opening of the cervix.

Oligohydramnios is a condition of low or missing amniotic fluid (olig/o = scanty + hydr/o = water, fluid + -amnios = amnion).

Polyhydramnios is a condition of excessive amniotic fluid.

Meconium is the term for the first feces of the newborn. If meconium staining occurs, it is fetal defecation while in utero and represents fetal distress. Meconium derives its name from the Greek term for poppy juice, which is a purplish-black color.

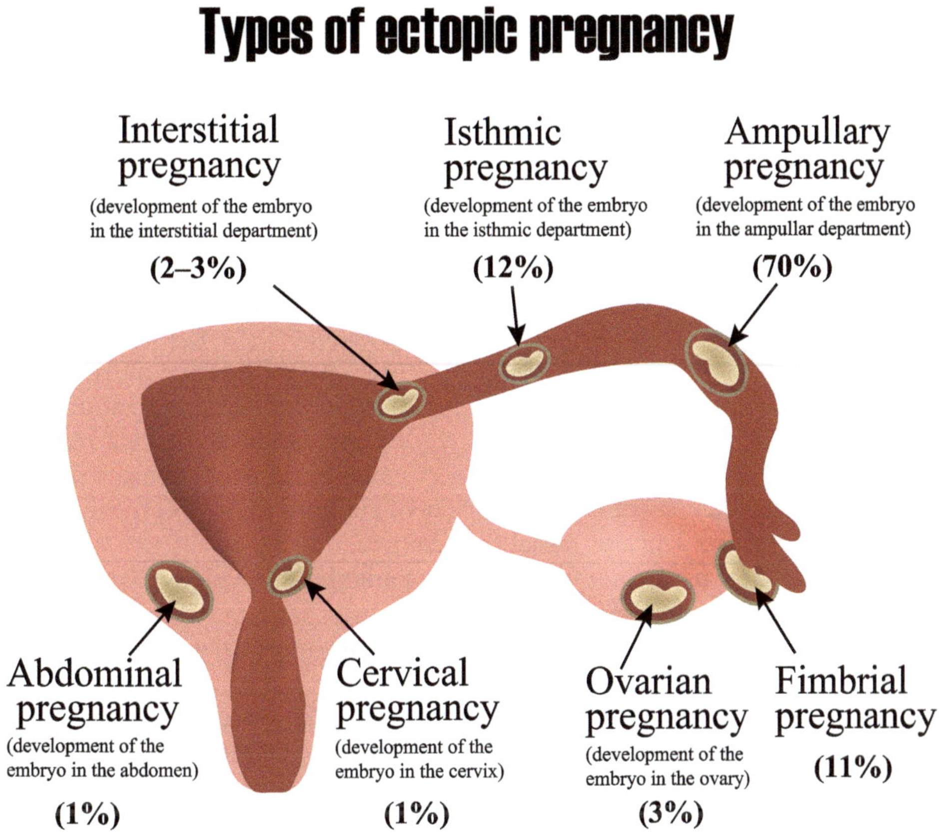

The presence of a nuchal cord is an abnormal but commonly occurrence in which the umbilical cord is wrapped around the neck of the neonate.

An Apgar score is an examination that uses a set of criteria to rate the physical health of the infant 1 and 5 minute after birth.

A congenital hypothyroidism test is conducted to detect deficient hormones. If undiscovered and not treated, this lack of hormones can lead to retarded growth and brain development.

A test for phenylketonuria seeks to detect a deficiency of the enzyme phenylalanine hydroxylase, which is responsible for converting phenylalanine, found in certain foods, into tyrosine. Failure to treat this condition will lead to brain damage and mental retardation.

An episiotomy is an incision to widen the vaginal opening (orifice) to prevent tearing of the tissue of the vulva during delivery. Decode and define the term *mediolateral*.

Oxytocia and dystocia are not really interventions, but are causes of concern. Oxytocia (oxy- = rapid + -tocia means labor, delivery). Dystocia is a difficult labor. The term eutocia (eu- means healthy or normal) is a normal, healthy delivery.

A vaginal birth after C-section (VBAC) is the delivery of an infant vaginally after a C-section.

A cephalic presentation (cephal/o = head) is the delivery of the baby head first, which is a usual, normal method. A breech delivery is a presentation that is feet or buttocks first and can be the reason for a C-section.

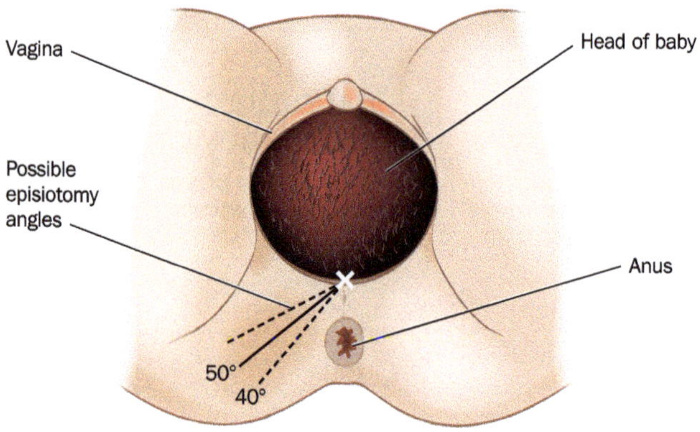

© Blamb/Shutterstock.com

A salpingosalpingostomy is a rejoining of previously cut fallopian tube to reestablish patency (openness). This is a reversal of a tubal ligation, similar to a vasovasostomy.

Sterilization is a surgical procedure of rendering a person unable to produce children. For women, this could be a hysterectomy, a bilateral oophorectomy, or a tubal ligation.

A tubal ligation is the cutting, tying (ligation), and cauterization (burning) the fallopian tubes to prevent released ova from being fertilized by spermatozoa.

Contraceptive management encompasses a variety of methods to control the time of pregnancy.

Abstinence is the total avoidance of sexual intercourse.

The rhythm method is a natural family planning method that involves charting the menstrual cycle to recognize fertile and infertile periods.

Barrier methods are different ways of preventing the physical union of an ovum and a spertmatozoon.

The contraceptive sponge is an intravaginal barrier with a spermicidal additive.

A diaphragm is a soft, rubber hemisphere that fits over the cervix to prevent sperm from entering.

Cervical caps are small rubber cups that fit over the cervix to prevent sperm from entering.

Male condoms are soft, flexible sheaths that cover the penis and prevent the sperm from entering the vagina.

Female condoms are soft, flexible sheaths that fit within the vagina and prevent sperm from entering the vagina.

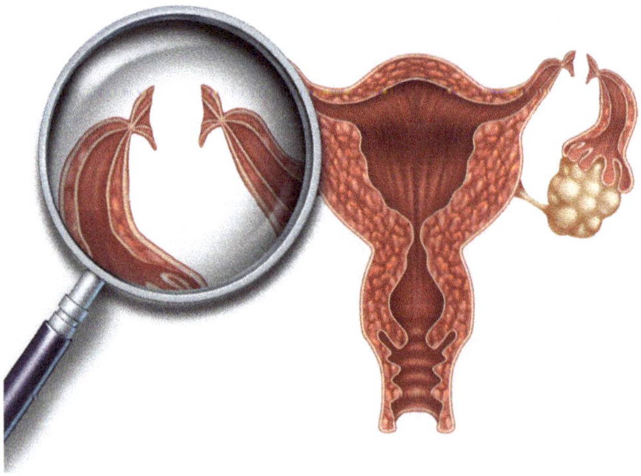
© Lightspring/Shutterstock.com

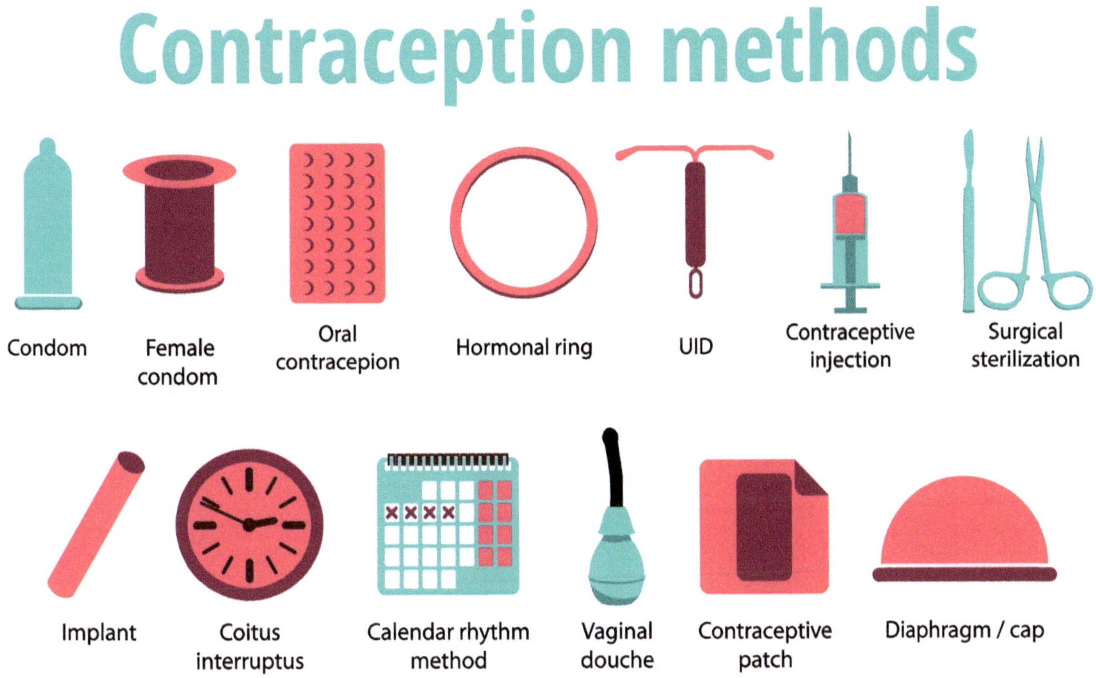

Abortifacients are medications that terminate pregnancy. Examples are mifepristone (Mifeprex) and dinoprostone (Prostin E2).

Emergency contraceptive pills (ECP) are medications that can prevent pregnancy after unprotected vaginal intercourse. It does not affect existing pregnancies or cause abortions. Plan B is a popular brand-name available ECP that in now available OTC.

CHAPTER 14

Eyes and Ears

The eye is made up of special anatomical structures that work together to facilitate sight. Light passes through the cornea, pupil, lens, and vitreous body to stimulate sensory receptors in the retina. Vision is made possible through the coordinated actions of nerves that control the movement of the eyeball.

The ear is described as having three divisions: the external ear, the middle ear, and the inner ear. The ear contains structures for both the sense of hearing and the sense of balance. The eights cranial nerve carries nerve impulses for both hearing and balance from the ear to the brain.

General combining forms for vision are opt/o and optic/o. Combining forms for hearing are audi/o and acous/o.

An ophthalmologist (ophthalm/o = eye + -logist = one who specializes in the study of) is one who specializes in the diagnosis and treatment of disorders and diseases of the eye. The discipline is called ophthalmology. Note that an ophthalmologist is an MD for eye disorders.

An optometrist (opt/o = vision + -metrist = one who specializes in measurement) is a specialist who measures your vision and prescribes corrective solutions as needed. Glasses and contact lenses used to be the main sources of correction; however, surgery is now becoming more of an option.

An audiologist (audi/o = hearing + -logist = one who specializes in the study of) is the healthcare specialist in the diagnosis, treatment, and prevention of hearing disorders. The specialist is an audiologist.

An otorhinolaryngologist (ot/o = ear + rhin/o = nose + laryng/o = voice box + -logist = one who specializes in the study of) is a medical doctor who specializes in the disorders of the ear, nose, and throat. The specialty is otorhinolaryngology.

Vision is accomplished through the eyeball and its adnexa. Use the diagram to explain the names for the parts listed.

The protective, bony socket that holds the eye is called the orbit.

The eyebrows mark the area above the orbit (supraorbital) and help keep the sun and perspiration from getting in one's eyes.

The corners of the eyes are called the canthi (s. canthus). The lateral canthus is the outer corner and the medial canthus is the corner that is closer to the nose.

The area in which the upper and lower eyelids close is called the palpebral fissure. Palpebr/o and blephar/o are combining forms for the eyelids. The term "fissure" is used throughout medical terminology to mean a deep slit, whether it is between the eyelids, in the skin, or on a bone. The act of blinking is called palpebration, obviously derived from one of the combining forms. Be careful not to confuse palpebrate with palpate or palpitate.

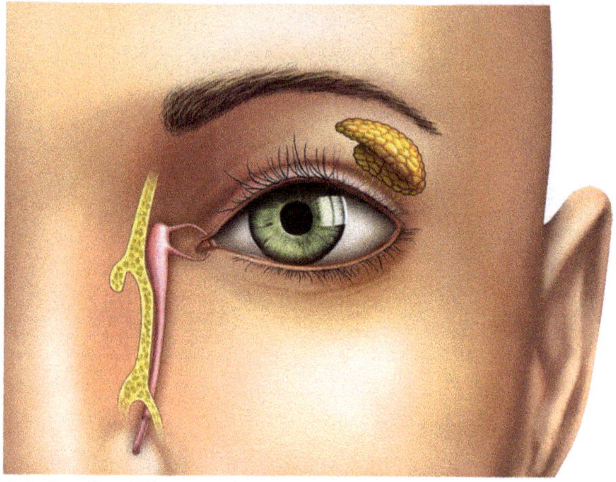

© Andrea Danti/Shutterstock.com

The thin protective mucous membrane that spreads to coat the anterior surface of the eyeball and the eyelids is called the conjunctiva (conjunctivae).

The eyeball is arranged in three layers/tunics. The outer layer/fibrous tunic is composed of the sclera and cornea. The sclera is the outermost lateral and posterior portion of the eye, referred to generally as the white of the eye. The portion of the sclera that covers the anterior section of the eye that is transparent is called the cornea. The border between the two is called the limbus.

Blepharedema (blephar/o = eyelid + -edema = swelling) is a swelling of the eyelid.

Blepharitis (blephar/o = eyelid + -itis = inflammation) is an inflammation of the eyelid.

Blepharochalasis (blephar/o = eyelid + -chalasis = relaxation, slackening) is a hypertrophy of the skin of the eyelid. *Point out that the upper image also is an example of blepharochalasis.*

Blepharoptosis (blephar/o = eyelid + -ptosis = drooping) is a drooping of the upper eyelid.

Ectropion (ec- = out + trop/o = turning + -ion = process of) is a turning outward (eversion) of the eyelid, exposing the conjunctiva.

Entropion (en- = in + trop/o = turning + -ion= process of) is a turning inward of the eyelid toward the eye.

Conjunctivitis (conjunctiv/o = conjunctiva + -itis = inflammation) is an inflammation of the conjunctiva, commonly known as the highly contagious disorder, pinkeye.

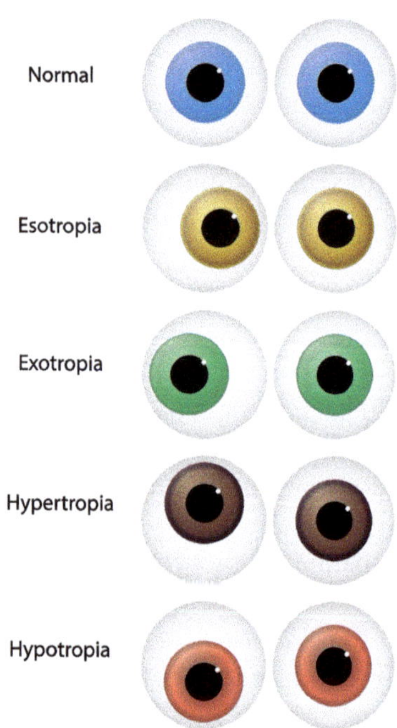

© Radu Bercan/Shutterstock.com

Ophthalmia neonatorum (ophthalm/o = eye + -ia = condition, neo- = new + nat/o = born + -um = structure) is a severe, purulent (characterized by pus) conjunctivitis in the newborn, usually due to gonorrheal or chlamydial infection. Routine introduction of an antibiotic ophthalmic ointment (erythromycin) prevents most cases.

Esotropia (eso- = inward + trop/o = turning + -ia = condition) is a turning inward of one or both eyes (cross eyes).

Exotropia (exo- = outward + trop/o = turning + -ia = condition) is a turning outward of one or both eyes.

Photophobia (phot/o = light + -phobia = condition of fear) is an extreme sensitivity to light, NOT a fear of light. Here, the word *fear* means an aversion.

A corneal ulcer is trauma to the outer covering of the eye resulting in an abrasion.

Keratitis (kerat/o = cornea + -itis = inflammation) is an inflammation of the cornea.

Aphakia (a- = without + phak/o = lens + -ia = condition) is a condition of no lens, either congenital or acquired.

A cataract is a progressive loss of transparency of the lens of the eye.

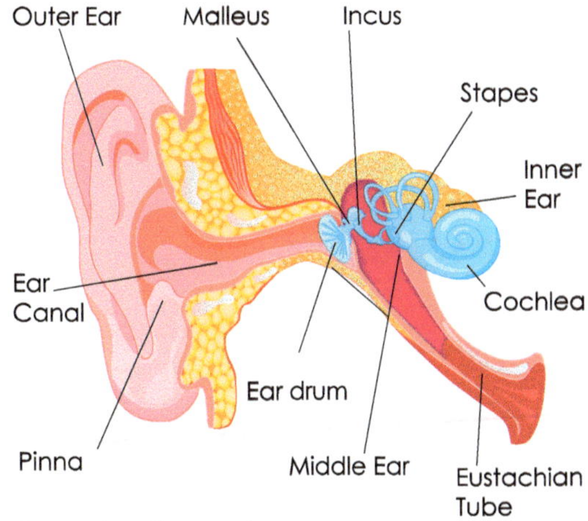

© snapgalleria/Shutterstock.com

Achromatopsia (a- = without, chromat/o = color + -opsia = vision condition) is an impairment of color vision. It is characterized by an inability to distinguish between certain colors because of abnormalities of the photopigments produced in the retina. It is commonly called color blindness.

Age-related macular degeneration (ARMD/AMD) is a progressive destruction of the macula, resulting in a loss of central vision. This is the most common visual disorder after the age of 75 years.

Intraocular melanoma (intra- = within + ocul/o = eye + -ar = pertaining to, melan/o = dark, black + -oma = tumor) is a malignant tumor of the choroid, ciliary body, or iris that usually occurs in individuals in their 50s or 60s.

A retinoblastoma (retin/o = retina + blast/o = embryonic, immature + -oma = tumor) is an inherited condition present at birth that arises from embryonic retinal cells.

The ear is divided into three parts: the outer, middle, and inner ear (also called the labyrinth).

Sound is conducted by air, bone, and fluid through these divisions. The majority of the ear is contained within the petrous (hard, stone-like) portion of the temporal bone.

Be careful! Do not confuse oral, meaning pertaining to the mouth, with aural, meaning pertaining to the ear.

The mastoid process is a hard, small projection of the temporal bone that is behind the opening of the auditory canal. Because of its proximity to the ear, it occasionally becomes involved with infections of the middle ear.

Otalgia (ot/o = ear + -algia and -dynia = pain) is an earache, pain in the ear. It is also called otodynia.

Otorrhea (ot/o = ear + -rrhea = discharge) is a discharge from the auditory canal; it may be serous (watery), bloody, or purulent (filled with pus).

Tinnitus is an abnormal sound heard in one or both ears and caused by trauma or disease. It may be a ringing, buzzing, or jingling. Make sure students realize that this is NOT an inflammation—the correct spelling is tinnit*us*, not tinnit*is*.

Vertigo is dizziness; there is an abnormal sensation of movement when there is no movement, either of oneself moving or of objects moving around oneself. It may be caused by middle ear infections or by the toxic effects of alcohol, sunstroke, and certain medications.

Otoscopy (ot/o = ear + -scopy = process of viewing) is a visual examination of the external auditory canal and the tympanic membrane using an instrument called an otoscope (ot/o = ear + -scope = instrument to view).

Tympanometry (tympan/o = eardrum + -metry = process of measuring) is the measurement of the condition and mobility function of the eardrum. The resultant graph is called a tympanogram (tympan/o = eardrum + -gram = a record, recording).

CHAPTER 15

Mental Health

Health is defined as a state of complete physical, mental, and social well-being, not just the absence of disease or infirmity. Mental health is a state of well-being in which the individual realizes his or her own abilities and can cope with the normal stressors of life and can make a contribution to society. Mental disorders are defined as an abnormal condition of the brain. It affects the way a person thinks, feels, behaves, and relates to others and to their surroundings. In many cases the exact cause of mental disorders is unknown.

Below are some interesting facts regarding mental health:

25% of Americans are diagnosed with a mental disorder
More than 25% of the top 100 medications prescribed are psychiatric drugs
Approximately 40 million Americans are diagnosed with anxiety
The fourth most common diagnostic category for inpatient admissions is substance-related mental disorders

Behavioral health reflects an integration of the interaction between mind and body. Behavior is observable and measurable.

A psychologist (psych/o = mind + -logist = one who specializes in the study of) is a healthcare professional who works with the diagnosis and treatment of mental health disorders. Psychology is the study of the mind.

A psychiatrist is a medical doctor who specializes in the treatment of mental disorders. The psychiatrist can prescribe medications (as a medical doctor), while the psychologist cannot. The discipline of psychiatrists is psychiatry.

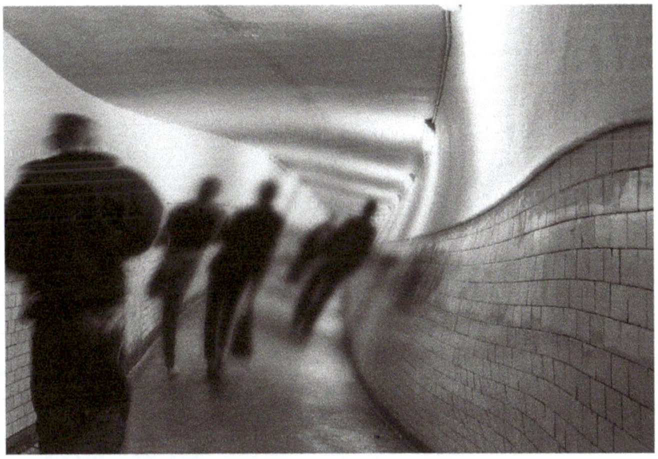
© ysuel/Shutterstock.com

A delusion is a persistent belief in a demonstrable untruth or a provable inaccurate perception despite clear evidence to the contrary.

A hallucination is any unreal sensory perception that occurs with no external cause.

An illusion is an inaccurate sensory perception based on a real stimulus; examples

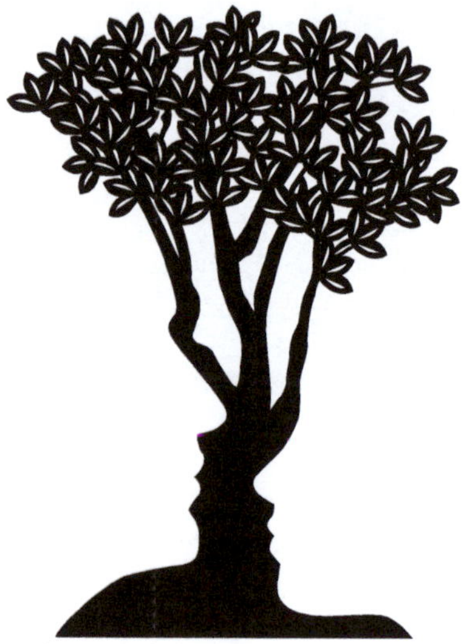

© Christos Georghiou/Shutterstock.com

include mirages and interpreting music or wind as voices (think of the mirages of water in the desert).

Confabulation is an effort to conceal a gap in memory by fabricating detailed, often believable stories. It is usually associated with alcohol abuse.

Defense mechanisms are unconscious mechanisms for psychological coping, adjustment, or self-preservation in the face of stress or a threat. Examples include denial of an unpleasant situation or condition and projection of intolerable aspects onto another individual.

Delirium is a condition of confused, unfocused, irrational agitation. In mental disorders, agitation and confusion may also be accompanied by a more intense disorientation, incoherence, or fear, and illusions, hallucinations, and delusions.

Dementia is a progressive loss of memory, personality alterations, confusion, loss of touch with reality, and stupor (seeming unawareness of, and disconnection with, one's surroundings).

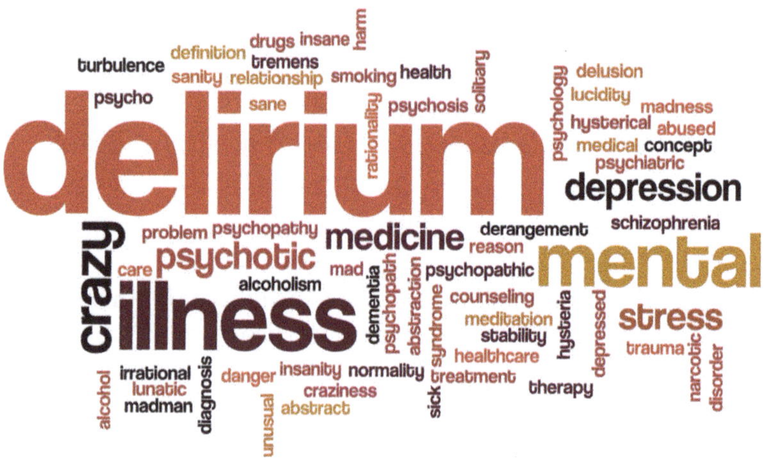

© ibreakstock/Shutterstock.com

Echolalia (echo- reverberation + -lalia = condition of babbling) is a repetition of words or phrases spoken by others.

Libido is a normal psychological impulse drive associated with sensuality, expressions of desire, or creativity. Abnormality occurs only when such drives are excessively heightened or depressed.

Psychosis (psych/o = mind + -osis = abnormal condition) is a dissociation with or impaired perception of reality. It may be

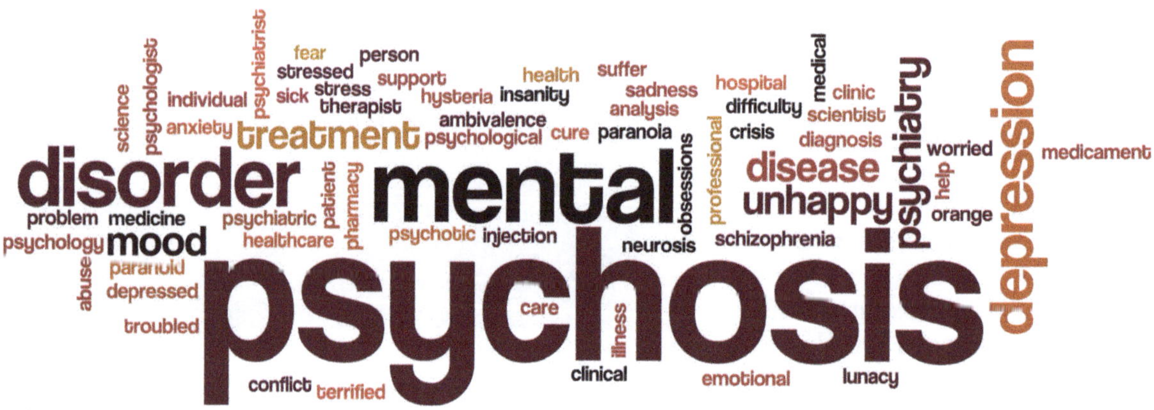

© ibreakstock/Shutterstock.com

accompanied by hallucinations, delusions, incoherence, akathisia, and/or disorganized behavior.

Somnambulism (somn/o = sleep + ambul/o = walking + -ism = condition) is the medical term for sleepwalking.

An affect is an observable demonstration of emotion that can be described in terms of quality, range, and appropriateness. Common examples of conditions of affect are:

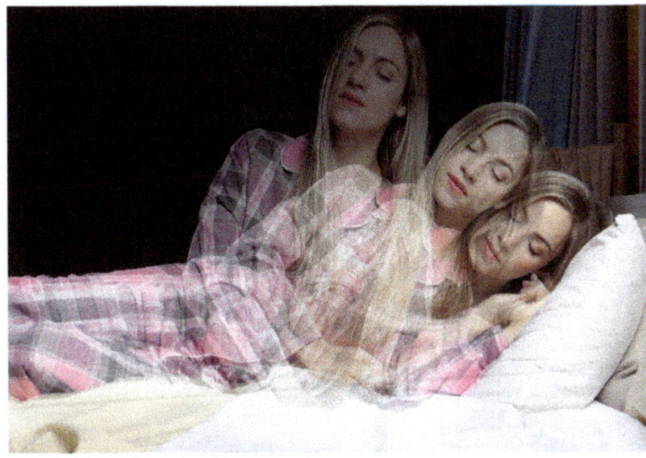

© Africa Studio/Shutterstock.com

- Blunted: a moderately reduced range of affect.
- Flat: a greatly decreased or a complete loss of emotional expression. It may be seen in schizophrenia, mental retardation, and some depressive disorders.
- Labile: multiple, abrupt changes in affect. It is seen in schizophrenia and bipolar disorder.
- Full/wide range: a generally appropriate emotional response.

Anxiety is an anticipation of impending change and dread accompanied by restlessness, tension, tachycardia (rapid heartbeat), and breathing difficulty not associated with an apparent stimulus.

Dysphoria (dys-= abnormal + -phor/o = to carry, to bear) is a generalized negative mood characterized by depression.

Euphoria (eu- = good, well) is an exaggerated sense of physical and emotional well-being not based on reality, disproportionate to the cause, or inappropriate to the situation.

Euthymia (eu- = good, well + -thymia = condition of the mind) is a normal range of moods and emotions.

Tourette syndrome is a group of involuntary behaviors that include the vocalization of words or sounds (sometimes obscene) and repetitive movements; it is a vocal and multiple tic disorder.

Conduct disorders are characterized by patterns of persistent aggressive and defiant behaviors. Oppositional defiant disorder (ODD) is characterized by hostile, disobedient behavior.

PDD is a group of developmental disorders characterized by impairment of communication skills and social interaction.

Asperger disorder is one of the psychological disorders that is first diagnosed in childhood. It is characterized by an impairment of social interaction and repetitive patterns of inappropriate behavior.

Autistic disorder (auto- = self + -istic = pertaining to) is a condition of an abnormal development of social interaction, impaired communication including delayed language acquisition, and repetitive

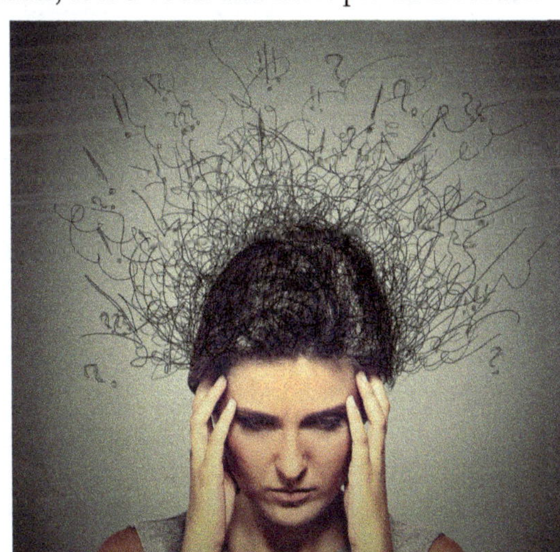

© pathdoc/Shutterstock.com

behaviors. It originally got its name from the fact that the individual appeared to be more absorbed in his or her own inner world than in his or her place in a social world that included others.

Rett disorder is characterized by initial normal functioning followed by a loss of social and intellectual functioning.

IQ stands for intelligence quotient, a measure of an individual's intellectual functioning compared to that of the general population.

Mental retardation is a condition of subaverage intellectual ability, along with impairments in social and educational functioning. Mental retardation is divided into the following levels:

- Mild mental retardation: IQ range of 50–69; learning difficulties result.
- Moderate mental retardation: IQ range of 35–49; support is needed to function in society.
- Severe mental retardation: IQ range of 20–34; continuous support is needed to live in society.
- Profound mental retardation: IQ less than 20; there are severe self-care limitations.

Substance abuse disorders are on the rise and include alcohol, tobacco, stimulants (including caffeine), inhalants, opioids, hallucinogens, cocaine, etc.

Acute intoxication (in- = in + toxic/o = poison + -ation = process of) is an episode of behavioral disturbance following ingestion of alcohol or psychotropic drugs.

Delirium tremens (DTs) is an acute and sometimes fatal delirium induced by the cessation of ingesting excessive amounts of alcohol over a long period of time.

Dependence syndrome is difficulty in controlling the use of a drug.

Harmful use is a pattern of drug use that causes damage to a person's health.

Tolerance is a state in which a body becomes accustomed to the substances ingested; hence the user requires greater amounts to create the desired effect.

A withdrawal state is a group of symptoms that occurs during cessation of the use of a regularly taken drug.

Acute and transient psychotic disorders are a heterogeneous group of disorders characterized by the acute onset of psychotic symptoms, such as delusions, hallucinations, and perceptual disturbances, and by the severe disruption of ordinary behavior.

- Acute onset is defined as a crescendo from a normal perceptual state to a clearly abnormal clinical picture in about 2 weeks or less. For these disorders, there is no evidence of organic causation. Perplexity and puzzlement are often present, but disorientation to time, place, and person is not persistent or severe enough to justify a diagnosis of organically caused delirium. The disorder may or may not be associated with acute stress (usually defined as stressful events preceding the onset by 1 or 2 weeks).

Persistent delusional disorders are a variety of disorders in which long-standing delusions constitute the only, or the most conspicuous, clinical characteristic and cannot be classified as organic, schizophrenic, or affective.

Schizophrenia (schiz/o = split + phren/o = mind + -ia = condition) is a series of disorders that are characterized by fundamental distortions of thinking and perception, coupled with affects that are inappropriate or blunted. The patient exhibits a characteristic inability to recognize an appropriate perception of reality. The patient's intellectual capacity is usually intact. Symptoms may include hallucinations, delusions, and thought disorders. Be careful! The combining form phren/o can mean mind or diaphragm.

Catatonic schizophrenia is dominated by prominent psychomotor disturbances that may alternate between extremes, such as hyperkinesis and stupor, and may be accompanied by a dreamlike (oneiric) state and hallucinations.

Disorganized schizophrenia is characterized by prominent affective changes, fleeting and fragmentary delusions and hallucinations, and irresponsible and unpredictable behavior. A shallow, inappropriate mood, flighty thoughts, social isolation, and incoherent speech are also present.

Paranoid schizophrenia is dominated by relatively stable, persistent delusions, usually accompanied by auditory hallucinations and perceptual disturbances in affect, volition (will), and speech.

Schizotypal disorder, although sometimes described as borderline schizophrenia, has none of the characteristic schizophrenic anomalies. Patients may exhibit anhedonia, eccentric behavior, cold affect, and social isolation.

Depressive disorder (depression) is typically characterized by its degree (minimal, moderate, severe) or number of occurrences (single or recurrent, persistent). Patients who are depressed exhibit dysphoria, a reduction of energy, and a decrease in activity. Symptoms include anhedonia, lack of an ability to concentrate, and fatigue. Patients may experience parasomnias (abnormal sleep patterns), diminished appetite, and loss of self-esteem.

Dysthymia (dys- = difficult + -thymia = condition of the mind) is a mild, chronic depression of mood that lasts for years but is not severe enough to justify a diagnosis of depression.

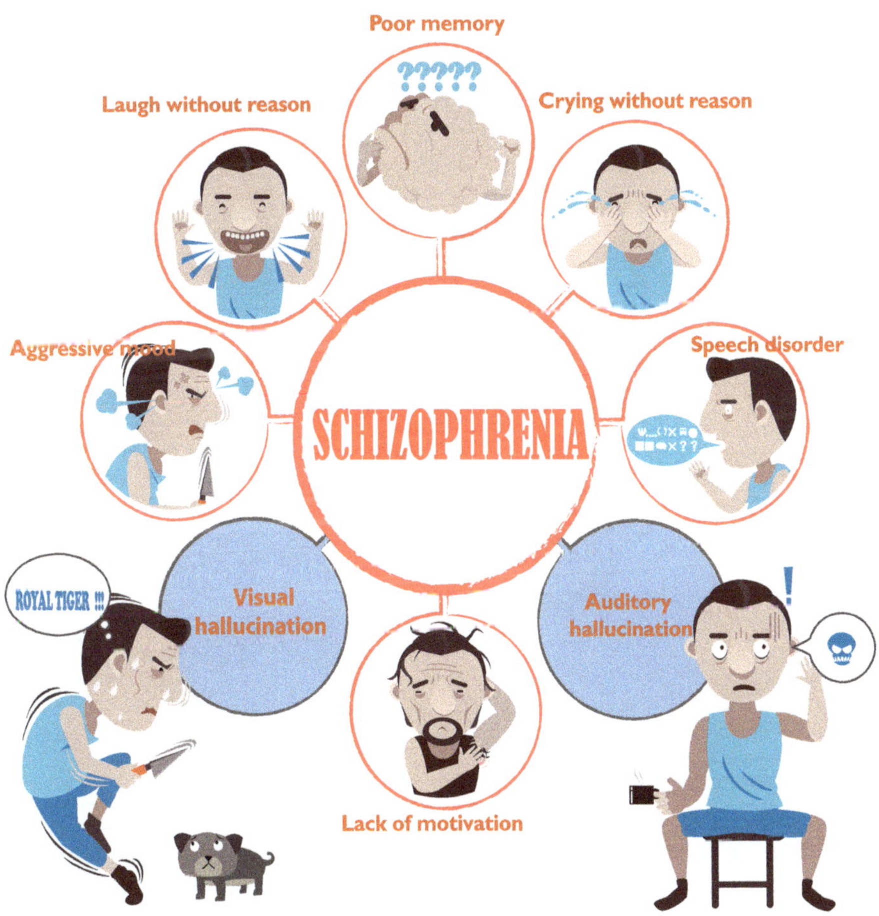

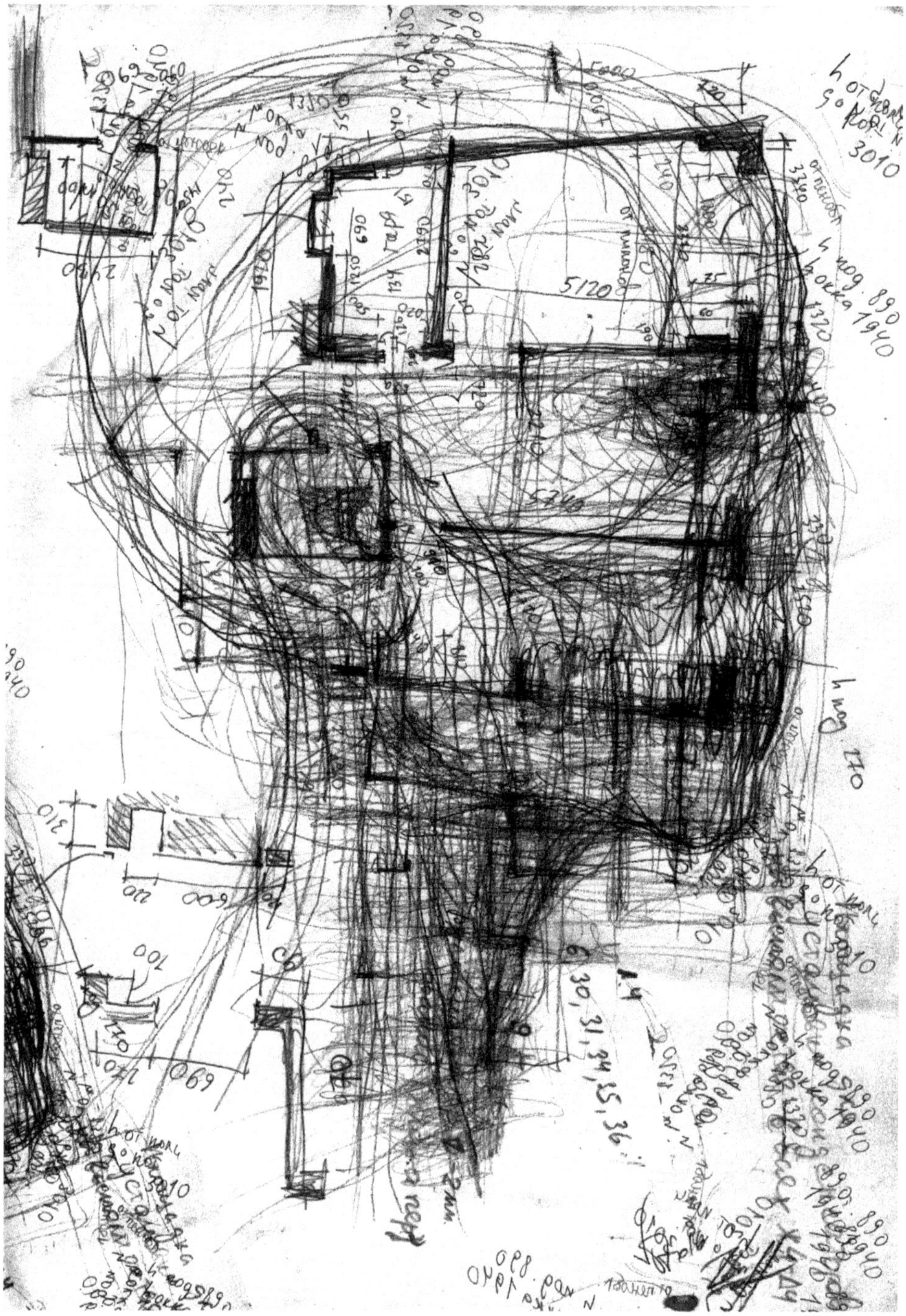

© Barandash Karandashich/Shutterstock.com

Hypomania (hypo- = decreased + -mania = condition of madness) is a disorder characterized by an inappropriate elevation of mood that may include positive and negative aspects. The patients may report increased feelings of well-being, energy, and activity, but may also report irritability and conceit.

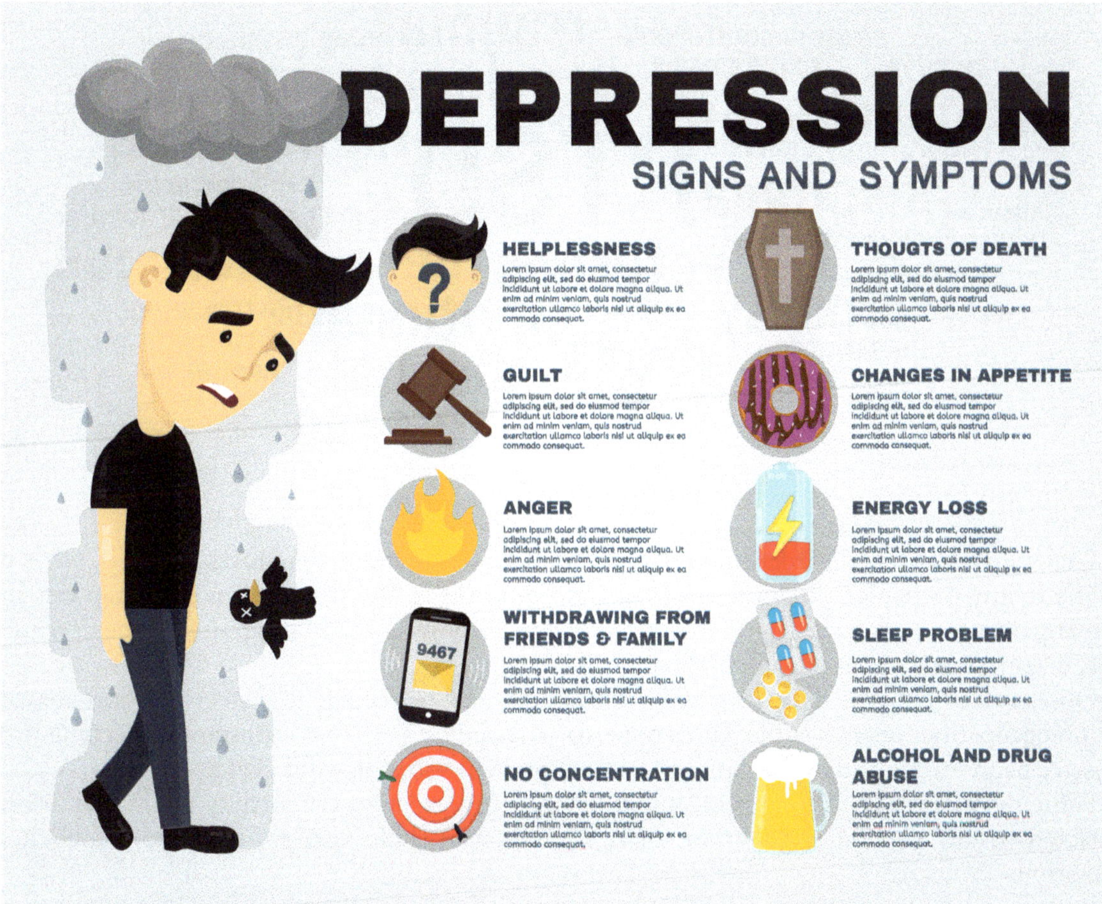

© svtdesign/Shutterstock.com

Bipolar disorder (BP) is a disorder characterized by swings between an elevation of mood and increased energy and activity (hypomania and mania) and a lowering of mood and decreased energy and activity (depression).

Cyclothymia (cycl/o = recurring) is a mood disorder characterized by recurring episodes of mild elation and depression that are not severe enough to warrant a diagnosis of bipolar disorder.

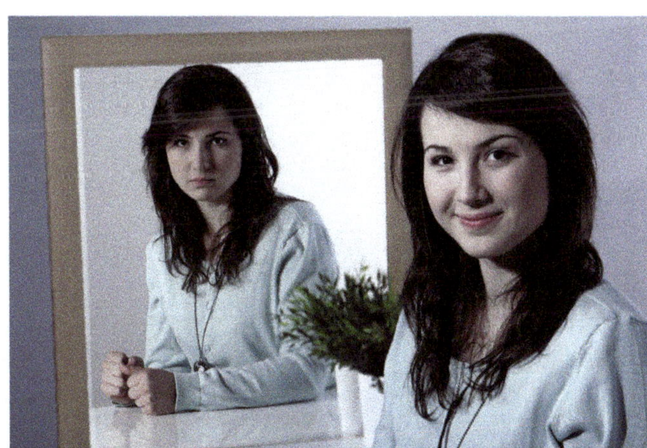

© Photographee.eu/Shutterstock.com

Seasonal affective disorder (SAD) is a weather-induced depression resulting from decreased exposure to sunlight in autumn and winter.

Persistent mood disorders are a group of long-term cyclic mood disorders in which the majority of the individual episodes are not sufficiently severe to warrant being described as hypomanic or mild depressive episodes.

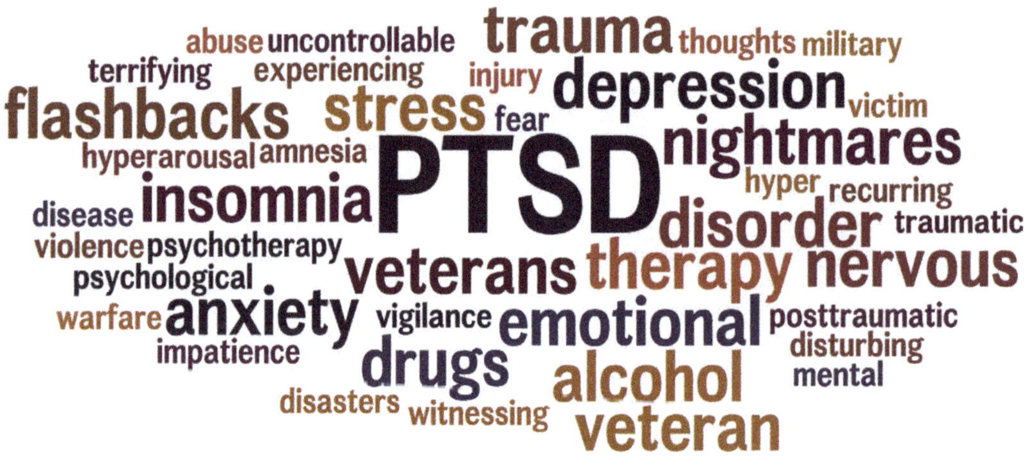

© serato/Shutterstock.com

Generalized anxiety disorder (GAD) is one of the most common diagnoses assigned, but is not specific to any particular situation or circumstance. GAD is NOT an acronym. Symptoms may include persistent nervousness, trembling, muscular tensions, sweating, lightheadedness, palpitations, dizziness, and epigastric discomfort.

Obsessive-compulsive disorder (OCD) is characterized by recurrent, distressing, and unavoidable preoccupations or irresistible drives to perform specific rituals (e.g., constantly checking locks, excessive hand washing) that the patient feels will prevent some harmful event.

Panic disorder (PD) is recurrent, unpredictable attacks of severe anxiety panic that are not restricted to any particular situation. Symptoms may include vertigo, chest pain, and heart palpitations.

Posttraumatic stress disorder (PTSD) is an extended emotional response to a traumatic event. Posttraumatic pertains to after (post-) trauma. The symptoms may include flashbacks, recurring nightmares, anhedonia, insomnia, hypervigilance, anxiety, depression, suicidal thoughts, and emotional blunting.

Anorexia (an- = without + orex/o = appetite + -ia = condition) nervosa is a prolonged refusal to eat adequate amounts of food and an altered perception of what constitutes a normal minimum weight caused by an intense fear of becoming morbidly obese. This disorder primarily affects adolescent females, but can affect males and other age groups as well. The disorder results in emaciation and amenorrhea.

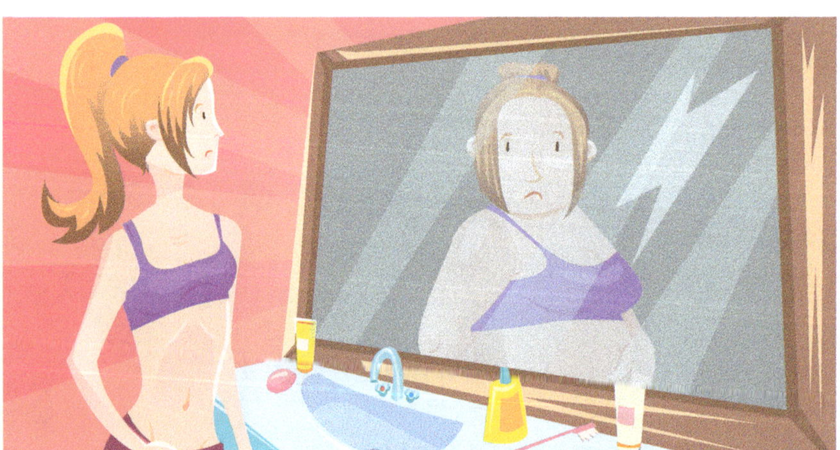
© movaliz/Shutterstock.com

Bulimia nervosa is an eating disorder in which

the individual eats large quantities of food and then purges the body through self-induced vomiting or inappropriate use of laxatives.

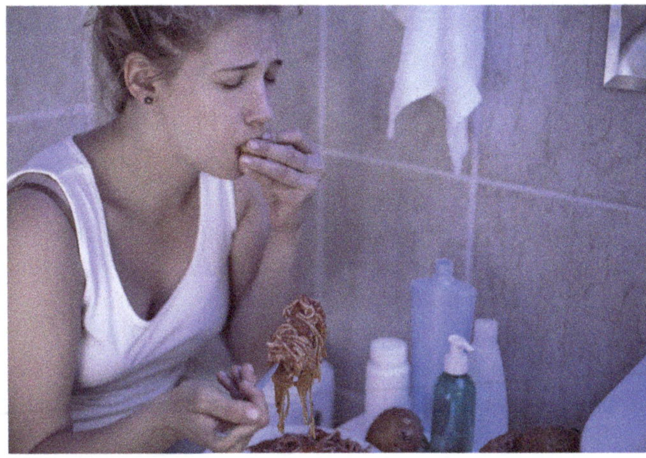

© Photographee.eu/Shutterstock.com

Anorexia has the highest mortality rate of any psychiatric disorder (7% to 24%)

Parasomnia (para- = abnormal + somn/o = sleep + -ia = condition) is an abnormal activation of physiologic functions during the sleep cycle. Examples include sleep terrors, in which repeated episodes of sudden awakening are accompanied by intense anxiety, agitation, amnesia, and somnambulism (sleepwalking).

Hypoactive sexual desire disorder is an indifference or unresponsiveness to sexual stimuli and an inability to achieve orgasm during intercourse.

Nymphomania (nymph/o = woman + -mania = condition of madness) is a relentless drive to achieve sexual orgasm in the female. In the male, the same condition is referred to as *satyriasis*.

Premature ejaculation is an involuntary, anxiety-induced ejaculation of semen during sexual activity.

Sexual anhedonia (an- = without + hedon/o = pleasure + -ia =condition) is an inability to enjoy sexual pleasure.

Kleptomania (klept/o = to steal + -mania = condition of madness) is an uncontrollable impulse to steal.

Pyromania (pyr/o = fire) is an uncontrollable impulse to set fires.

Trichotillomania (trich/o = hair + till/o = pulling) is an uncontrollable impulse to pull one's hair out by the roots.

Paraphilias (para- = abnormal + phil/o = attraction + -ia = condition) are literally abnormal attractions.

Pedophilia (ped/o) is a sexual preference, whether real or imagined, for children as a means of sexual gratification.

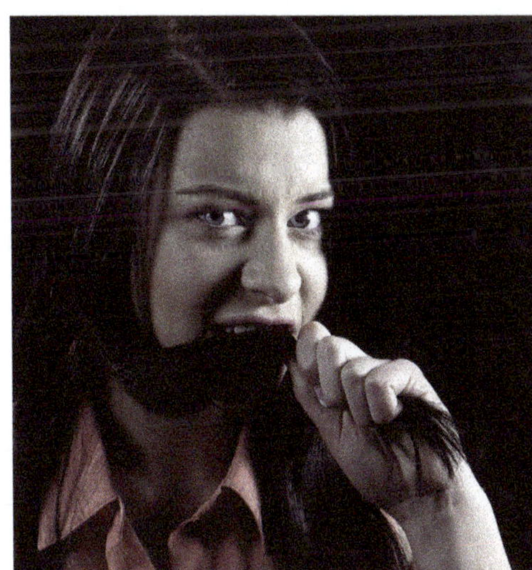

© Rebbeck Images/Shutterstock.com

Exhibitionism is a condition in which the patient derives sexual arousal from the exposure of his or her genitals to strangers.

Fetishism is reliance on an object as a stimulus for sexual arousal and pleasure.

Sadomasochism is preference for sexual activity that involves inflecting or receiving pain and/or humiliation.

Voyeurism is a condition in which an individual derives sexual pleasure and gratification from surreptitiously looking at individuals engaged in intimate behavior.

The DSM IV-TR multiaxial assessment diagnosis is a measure of the mental health of an individual across five axes. The first three (if named) are diagnostic codes. The fourth axis is a statement of factors influencing the patient's mental health (examples include lack of social supports, unemployment). The fifth axis is a numeral score that summarizes a patient's overall functioning.

A mental status examination is a diagnostic procedure to determine a patient's current mental state. It includes assessment of the patient's appearance, affect, thought processes, cognitive function, insight, and judgment.

Laboratory tests may be done to determine underlying pathology. Urinalyses with drug screens, blood alcohol levels, screening tests for syphilis, thyroid function panels, and complete blood counts with differential and blood chemistry are examples.

Imaging can be helpful to rule out neurologic disorders. Computed tomography and magnetic resonance imaging can be used to screen for brain lesions. Positron emission tomography scans can be used to examine and map the metabolic activity of the brain.

Behavioral therapy is a therapeutic attempt to alter an undesired behavior by substituting a new response or set of responses to a given stimulus.

Cognitive therapy is a wide variety of treatment techniques that attempt to help the individual to alter inaccurate or unhealthy perceptions and patterns of thinking.

Psychoanalysis is a behavioral treatment developed initially by Sigmund Freud to analyze and treat any dysfunctional effects of unconscious factors on a patient's mental state. This therapy uses techniques that include analysis of defense mechanisms and dream interpretation.

Detoxification is the removal of a chemical substance (drug or alcohol) as an initial step in the treatment of a chemically dependent individual.

Electroconvulsive therapy (ECT) is a method of inducing convulsions to treat affective disorders in patients who have been resistant or unresponsive to drug therapy.

Light therapy is the exposure of the body to light waves to treat patients with depression due to seasonal fluctuations.

Hypnosis is the induction of an altered state of consciousness to change an unwanted behavior or emotional response.

Narcosynthesis (narc/o = sleep, stupor + -synthesis = bringing together) is the use of intravenous barbiturates to elicit repressed memories or thoughts.

Pharmacotherapy is the use of medication to affect behavior or emotions.

www.ingramcontent.com/pod-product-compliance
Ingram Content Group UK Ltd.
Pitfield, Milton Keynes, MK11 3LW, UK
UKHW052008041026
15590UKWH00008B/2226

9 781524 921019

MEDICAL
TERMINOLOGY

JERRY S. FINDLEY

Kendall Hunt
publishing company

ISBN 978-1-5249-2101-9
90000
9 781524 921019